TABLE OF CONTENTS

PURPOSE OF REPORT

To accelerate the use of health information technology (IT), Congress passed and President Obama signed into law the Health Information Technology for Economic and Clinical Health (HITECH) Act as part of the American Recovery and Reinvestment Act of 2009. The HITECH Act authorized the Centers for Medicare & Medicaid Services (CMS) to provide financial incentives to eligible hospitals, Critical Access Hospitals (CAHs), and eligible professionals to adopt and meaningfully use certified electronic health record (EHR) technology to improve patient care.[1] The HITECH Act also authorized the Office of the National Coordinator for Health Information Technology (ONC) to establish and administer programs to guide physicians, hospitals, and other key entities as they adopt and meaningfully use certified EHR technology as established in subsequent federal regulations.

Section 13113(a) of the American Recovery and Reinvestment Act of 2009 under Title XIII of Division A, part of the HITECH Act requires a report to be submitted to Congress no later than two years after the enactment of the law, and annually thereafter. The Secretary of Health and Human Services submitted the first report on January 17, 2012. This report is the annual update to the previous submission.

This report provides: (1) updates on the adoption of health IT; (2) efforts of CMS and ONC to facilitate nationwide adoption and exchange of electronic health information; and, (3) identification and discussion of barriers to the adoption and exchange of electronic clinical data and how ONC's programs are addressing those barriers.

EXECUTIVE SUMMARY

OVERVIEW

Information is widely recognized as "the lifeblood of modern medicine."[2] Health information technology (health IT) has the potential to improve the flow of information across the health care system and serve as the infrastructure to enable care transformation.[3,4] Health IT comprises technologies — from electronic health records (EHRs) and personal health records (PHRs) to remote monitoring devices and mobile health applications — that can collect, store, and transmit health information. By enabling health information to be used more effectively and efficiently throughout our health system, health IT has the potential to empower providers and patients; make health care and the health system more transparent; enhance the study of care delivery and payment systems; and drive substantial improvements in care, efficiency, and population health.

ONC collaborates with policymakers and stakeholders to address critical issues related to health IT. Working directly with the health IT community, ONC develops consensus-based standards and technologies that facilitate interoperability and health information exchange (HIE). ONC aims to protect the privacy and security of health information and ensure the safe use of health IT in every phase of its development and implementation. The ultimate goal of these efforts is to inspire confidence and trust in health IT. ONC provides expertise, guidance, and resources to ensure that health IT is widely and effectively implemented. ONC also administers a reliable Health IT Certification Program and works closely with CMS to establish the certification criteria for certified EHR technology (CEHRT) that eligible providers must adopt and meaningfully use in order to qualify for incentive payments under the Medicare and Medicaid EHR Incentive Programs.

PROGRESS ON ADOPTION OF EHR TECHNOLOGY & E-PRESCRIBING

Data show steady increases in the adoption of EHRs and key computerized functionalities related to EHR Incentive Programs' Meaningful Use criteria among office-based physicians and non-federal acute care hospitals.

★ In 2012, nearly three-quarters of office-based physicians (72 percent) had adopted any EHR system. Forty percent of physicians have adopted a "basic" EHR with certain advanced capabilities, more than double the adoption rate in 2009.[5] Physicians achieved at least fifty percent adoption rates for 12 of the 15 EHR Incentive Programs' Stage 1 Meaningful Use core objectives.[6]

★ As of 2012, 44 percent of non-federal acute care hospitals had adopted a "basic" EHR, more than triple the adoption rate of 2009.[7] The percent of hospitals with certified EHR technology increased by 18 percent between 2011 and 2012, rising from 72 percent to 85 percent.[8] Hospital adoption rates for Meaningful Use Stage 1 requirements for the EHR Incentive Programs' ranged from 72 percent to 94 percent.[9]

★ The percent of physicians e-prescribing using an EHR on one of the nation's largest e-prescribing network (Surescripts) increased almost eight-fold from 7 percent in December 2008 to over half of physicians (54 percent) in December 2012.[10] In the same period, the percent of community pharmacies active on the Surescripts network grew from 69 percent to 95 percent. The percent of new and renewal prescriptions sent electronically between 2008 and 2012 has increased ten-fold to approximately 47 percent.

PROGRESS ON MEANINGFUL USE ATTAINMENT

The CMS Medicare and Medicaid EHR Incentive Programs provide financial incentives for the adoption and Meaningful Use of certified EHR technology to improve patient care. CMS established the EHR Incentive Programs through notice and comment rulemaking and created the necessary infrastructure to implement the program in accordance with existing payment policies and program eligibility criteria. CMS regulations spell out the objectives for the Meaningful Use requirements that eligible professionals, eligible hospitals, and CAHs must meet in order to receive an incentive payment.[11] In addition to the incentives, eligible professionals, eligible hospitals, and CAHs that fail to demonstrate Meaningful Use of certified EHR technology will be subject to payment adjustments under Medicare beginning in 2015.

As of April 2013, more than 291,000 professionals, representing more than half of the nation's eligible professionals, have received incentive payments through the EHR Incentive Programs. Over 3,800 hospitals, representing about 80 percent of eligible hospitals, and including Critical Access Hospitals, have received incentive payments through this program as well.

Key Programs and Offices involved with the adoption of Health IT

Centers for Medicare & Medicaid Services:

Office of eHealth Standards and Services (OESS): OESS coordinates agency eHealth efforts to share healthcare data freely and easily among patients, physicians, healthcare providers, and health plans to improve health outcomes and reduce costs. OESS administers the Medicare and Medicaid EHR Incentive Programs and is the agency lead for privacy policy and compliance. OESS coordinates initiatives to improve interoperability, including the standardization of operating rules and electronic transactions for healthcare billing and payment and preparation for the transition to using the ICD-10 code sets for improved capture of granular health care information for both billing and quality measurement reporting.

Office of Information Systems (OIS): OIS provides information technology and program management support for the EHR Incentive Programs. In addition to designing, developing, and maintaining several data repositories and interfaces, OIS manages and oversees the EHR Information Center, which responds to provider inquiries about the EHR Incentive Programs, manages system operations support, and oversees data quality and reporting.

Office of Financial Management (OFM): OFM determines provider eligibility for participation in the EHR Incentive Programs, generates and distributes the incentive payments and conducts pre and post payment audits to assure program integrity.

Centers for Medicaid and CHIP Services (CMCS): The Medicaid EHR Incentive Program eligibility and program policies are determined by CMCS in coordination with each state. CMCS plays a leadership role in the coordination within and among states to support the implementation of EHRs, and coordinates with state Medicaid program expansion and health marketplace efforts.

Centers for Clinical Quality and Standards (CCSQ): In order to reduce provider burden with regards to reporting, CMS has worked with partners and representatives from industry to identify and finalize a set of unified quality measures that eligible health care providers could report to satisfy some of the various requirements of multiple programs in addition to meeting EHR Incentive Programs clinical quality measures requirements, including the Physician Quality Reporting System. CCSQ also administers a number of quality reporting programs, including the eRx Incentive Program, which also encourages provider to electronically prescribe. CCSQ is working to implement a unified set of electronic clinical quality measures (eCQMs) and electronic reporting requirements in order to permit broad scale electronic reporting of quality data across CMS programs.

Center for Medicare and Medicaid Innovation (Innovation Center): The Innovation Center identifies, creates, tests, and evaluates new payment and service delivery models to reduce program expenditures while preserving or enhancing the quality of care furnished to Medicare, Medicaid, and Children's Health Insurance Program (CHIP) beneficiaries. Several of the Innovation Center's models are testing the use of health IT in payment and payment and service delivery models, including the Health Care Innovation Awards and Pioneer Accountable Care Organizations models.

The Office of the National Coordinator for Health IT:

Health IT Regional Extension Centers Program (REC): RECs have played a pivotal role in providing technical assistance to providers. The 62 RECs are actively working with over 133,000 primary care providers, surpassing the 2012 HHS High Priority Goal of providing assistance to 100,000 primary care providers.

State Health Information Exchange (HIE) Program: The State HIE Program is responsible for coordinating the efforts of states to offer providers a variety of mechanisms to exchange health information electronically and developing governance mechanisms to ensure the efficient exchange of health information.

Workforce Development Program: The program's goal is to train a new workforce of skilled health IT professionals to help providers implement EHRs and achieve Meaningful Use. As of January 2013, the Community College Consortia Program has trained over 17,000 professionals and the University-Based Training Program has trained 983 professionals.

Beacon Community Program: The program supports 17 communities located throughout the U.S. in their goal of translating health IT investments and Meaningful Use of certified EHR technology to advance the vision of patient-centered care, while improving the quality of care and lowering costs.

Office of Certification (OCERT): OCERT authorizes the certification bodies that assess health IT that has been successfully tested by an accredited test lab to ensure it meets the functional requirements for certification. Providers participating in the Medicare and Medicaid EHR Incentive Programs must demonstrate Meaningful Use of certified EHR technology to earn the incentive payments. As of February 2013, 937 vendors had sought certification for 3,052 EHR technology products.

Office of the Chief Privacy Officer (OCPO): OCPO develops and coordinates privacy, security, and data stewardship policy with the HHS Office for Civil Rights and across the federal government, state and regional agencies, and foreign countries by providing subject matter expertise and technical support.

Office of Science and Technology (OST): OST promotes the development and implementation of interoperability standards and interoperable, standards-based technologies and open architectures that allow information to flow seamlessly and securely between health IT products. By engaging a range of stakeholders through a standardized framework, OST accelerates the development and harmonization of health IT standards that meet the needs of the health care provider, public health, and health IT vendor communities.

Office of Consumer e-Health (OCEH): OCEH works to empower patients and caregivers to be partners in their health care through the adoption and use of health IT. The office has expanded consumers' access to their electronic health information through outreach and support to health care organizations to provide patients the ability to view and download their health information via the "Blue Button."

Office of the Chief Medical Officer (OCMO): OCMO engages clinicians toward the Meaningful Use of certified EHR technology, coordinates the development of tools and resources for health IT-enabled quality improvement including clinical quality measures (CQM) and clinical decision support interventions (CDS), and works with stakeholders to assure that health IT enhances patient safety, and that health IT systems are usable and safe.

BARRIERS TO ADOPTION OF HEALTH INFORMATION TECHNOLOGY

Despite recent progress in increasing the adoption of health IT, providers still face challenges. The top barriers to EHR adoption reported by office-based physicians include the cost of purchasing an EHR system and concerns regarding loss of productivity. At least 4 in 10 physicians who have yet to adopt EHRs also express concerns regarding EHR maintenance costs, selecting an EHR that meets their practice's needs, adequacy of technical support, and practice resistance.[12] Key HITECH programs address many of these barriers, including the EHR Incentive Programs that offer financial incentives that support adoption and Meaningful Use of certified EHR technology and the REC Program that helps providers adopt and make Meaningful Use of EHRs. In order to address potential barriers to adoption related to privacy and security of electronic health information, the Office of the Chief Privacy Officer in ONC has developed a flexible, iterative process for assessing, prioritizing, and implementing privacy- and security-related initiatives.

Based upon the data that are currently available, which in some cases is dated, adoption of computerized technology varies across providers ineligible for the EHR Incentive Program. This report also describes barriers to EHR adoption and examples of efforts to support health IT adoption among these providers.

While recent years have seen a dramatic increase in the number of U.S. providers using health IT, expanding interoperability remains a challenge. Enabling exchange will involve reducing the cost and complexity of electronic health information exchange, ensuring trust among the key participants of exchange and encouraging exchange of information, particularly during transitions of care. ONC is playing a central role in enabling each of these key goals. The State HIE Program grantees have taken a variety of approaches to address these goals, examples of which are described in this report. Stage 2 Meaningful Use requirements for the EHR Incentive Programs has key criteria related to health information exchange that will enable exchange of key clinical information during transitions of care and ensure that providers can exchange information with others, regardless of EHR vendor. A recent Request for Information (RFI) that ONC developed in conjunction with CMS seeks specific suggestions on how to expand interoperability, including a combination of incentives, payment adjustments, and requirements that will lead to a more coordinated, value-driven health care system.

Additionally, ONC's work on developing standards may also help reduce the cost and complexity of exchange, while ONC's efforts to ensure the privacy and security of electronic health information helps promote trust in HIE among key participants. ONC also launched the Exemplar Health Information Exchange Governance Entities Program. This cooperative agreement program funded entities to advance and further develop existing health information exchange governance models. Strong governance can help ensure secure electronic health information exchange, reduce the cost and complexity of implementation, and assure the privacy and security of the electronic exchange of health information.

ADOPTION OF ELECTRONIC HEALTH RECORDS

Adoption of EHRs by both physicians and hospitals has increased substantially since the passage of the HITECH Act (Figures 1 and 2).[13,14] In 2009, approximately one in five office-based physicians and one in eight non-federal acute care hospitals had adopted a "basic" EHR with certain advanced capabilities. By 2012, adoption of "basic" EHRs doubled among physicians and tripled among hospitals; four in ten physicians and over four in ten hospitals had adopted a "basic" EHR system.

The EHR adoption measures reported in this chapter are based upon nationally representative surveys of office-based physicians and non-federal acute care hospitals and are not limited to eligible professionals and hospitals participating in the EHR Incentive Programs.

Key measures of adoption of EHR technology reported in this chapter are listed and described below.

- "Basic" EHR measures the adoption of specific capabilities that overlap but do not directly align with the EHR Incentive Programs' Meaningful Use objectives. An expert panel prior to HITECH selected these capabilities and it has been historically used to monitor trends in EHR adoption for both hospitals and physicians.[15]

- "Any" EHR measures the adoption of an EHR that is partially or fully electronic and provides a high-level overview of physicians' adoption of computerized technology. An equivalent measure is not available for hospitals.

- Adoption of certified EHRs that meet the EHR Incentive Programs' Meaningful Use objectives is available for hospitals but not currently available for physicians based upon national survey data.

- Physician and hospital adoption of individual electronic capabilities associated with EHR Incentive Programs' Meaningful Use objectives are available for many but not all the core objectives and only few of the menu objectives based upon national survey data.

- Statistics related to eligible professionals and hospitals attesting to Meaningful Use are reported in the next chapter.

Figure 1. Percentage of office-based physicians with EHRs: United States, 2008–2012

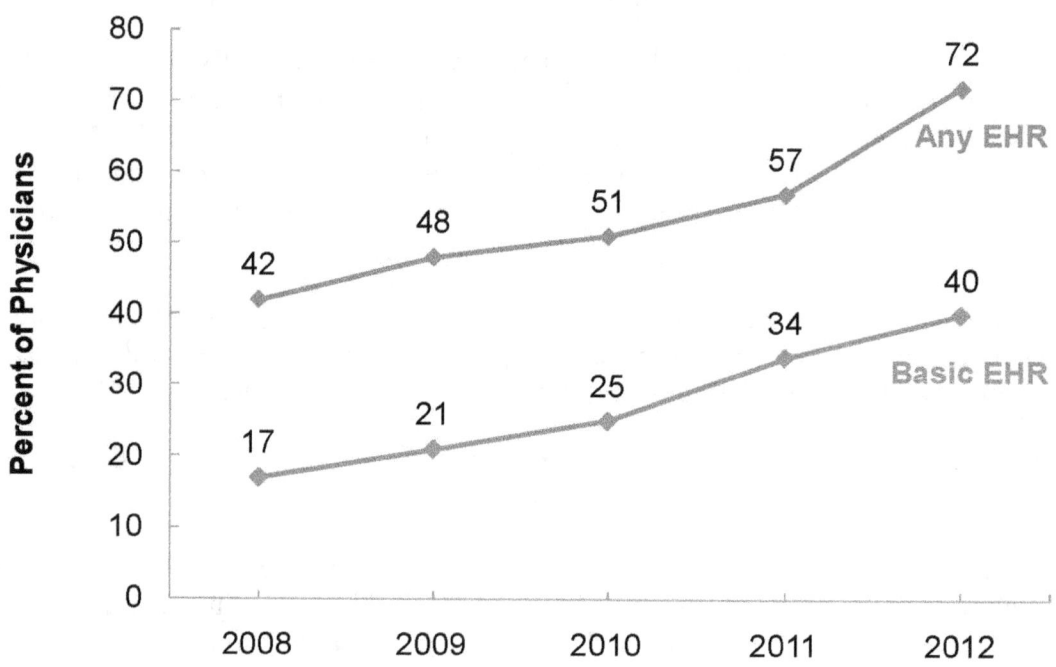

NOTES: "Any EHR system" is a medical or health record system that is all or partially electronic (excluding billing systems). A basic EHR includes: patient history and demographics, patient problem lists, physician clinical notes, comprehensive list of patients' medications and allergies, computerized orders for prescriptions, and view laboratory and imaging results electronically.
SOURCE: ONC analysis of the National Center for Health Statistics' 2008-2012 National Electronic Health Records Surveys.

★ In 2012, nearly three-quarters (72 percent) of office-based physicians adopted an EHR that was all or partially electronic, up from 42 percent in 2008 (Figure 1).

★ Between 2009 and 2012, the percentage of office-based physicians adopting a basic EHR system with certain advanced capabilities nearly doubled, growing from 21 percent to 40 percent.

Figure 2. Percent of non-federal acute care hospitals with adoption of at least a basic EHR system and possession of a certified EHR: 2008-2012

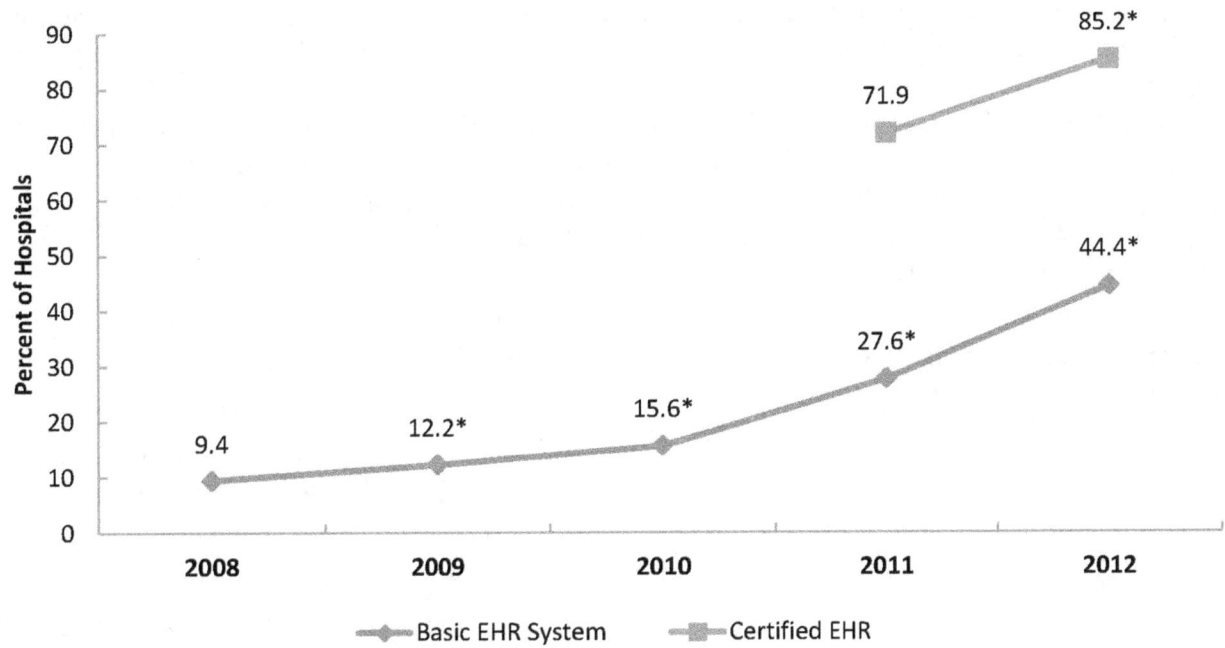

NOTES: Basic EHR adoption requires the EHR system to have at least a basic set of EHR functions, including clinician notes. A certified EHR is EHR technology that has been certified as meeting federal requirements for some or all of the hospital objectives of Meaningful Use. Possession means that the hospital has a legal agreement with the EHR vendor, but is not equivalent to adoption.
*Significantly different from previous year (p < 0.05).
SOURCE: ONC/American Hospital Association (AHA), AHA Annual Survey Information Technology Supplement

★ Hospital adoption of at least a basic EHR system with certain advanced capabilities more than tripled since 2009, increasing from 12 percent to 44 percent (Figure 2).

★ The percent of hospitals possessing certified EHR technology increased by 18 percent between 2011 and 2012, rising from 72 percent to 85 percent.

ADOPTION OF EHR TECHNOLOGY TO MEET MEANINGFUL USE OBJECTIVES

To participate in CMS' Medicare and Medicaid EHR Incentive Programs, eligible professionals and hospitals are required to demonstrate use of computerized capabilities of certified EHR technology that meet defined Meaningful Use objectives. Analyses of nationally representative survey of office-based physicians and non-federal acute care hospitals demonstrate strong and steady growth in both physician and hospital adoption of EHR technology to meet Meaningful Use objectives to improve quality, safety, and efficiency (Figures 3 and 4).[16,17] This suggests that EHRs that are being adopted possess advanced functionalities. As of 2012, half or more of physicians had the capability to meet 12 of the EHR Incentive Programs' Meaningful Use core objectives[i] (Figure 5 and 6) and hospital adoption rates for each of 14 Meaningful Use Stage 1 core objectives ranged from 72 percent to 94 percent (Table 1).

Figure 3. Percent of physicians with computerized capabilities to meet Meaningful Use core objectives: 2009-2012

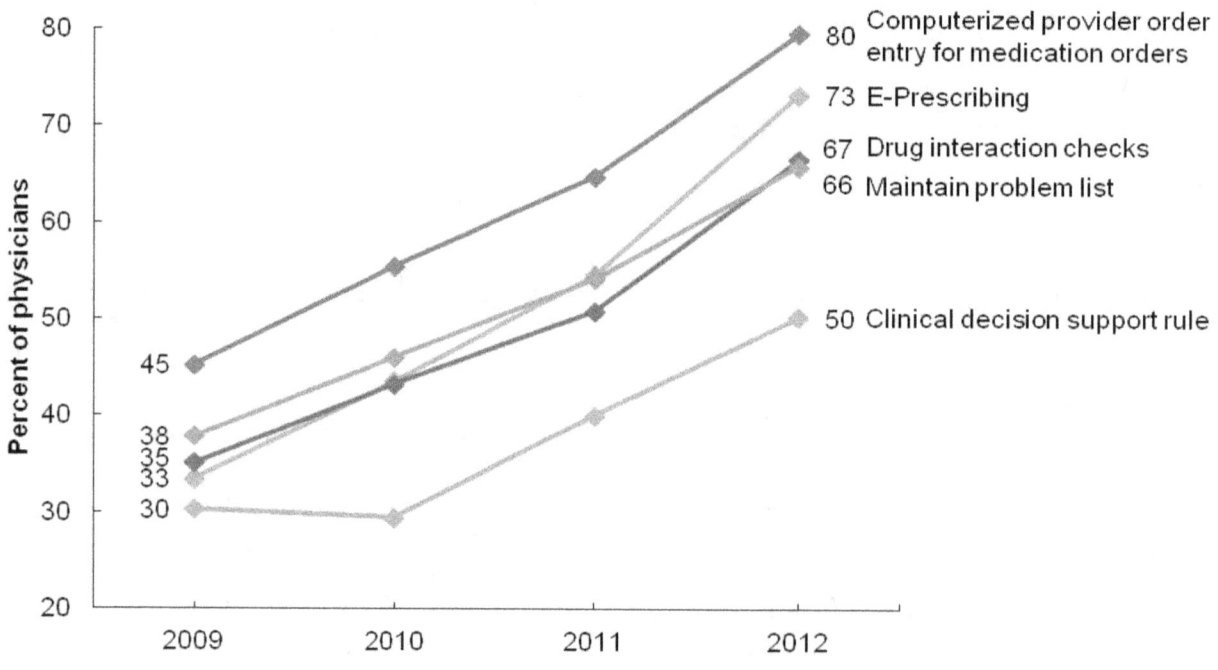

2012 is significantly different from 2009 for all computerized capabilities (p < 0.01).
SOURCE: ONC analysis of National Center for Health Statistics' 2009-2012 National Electronic Health Records Surveys.

★ Since HITECH was enacted, physician adoption of EHR technology to meet each of five EHR Incentive Programs' Meaningful Use core objectives has increased by at least 66 percent (Figure 3).

★ Since 2009, the percent of physicians with e-prescribing has more than doubled (119 percent increase).

---

[i] Data is only available for 12 of the 15 Meaningful Use core objectives.

Figure 4. Percent of non-federal acute care hospitals with computerized capabilities to meet selected EHR Incentive Programs' Meaningful Use objectives: 2008-2012

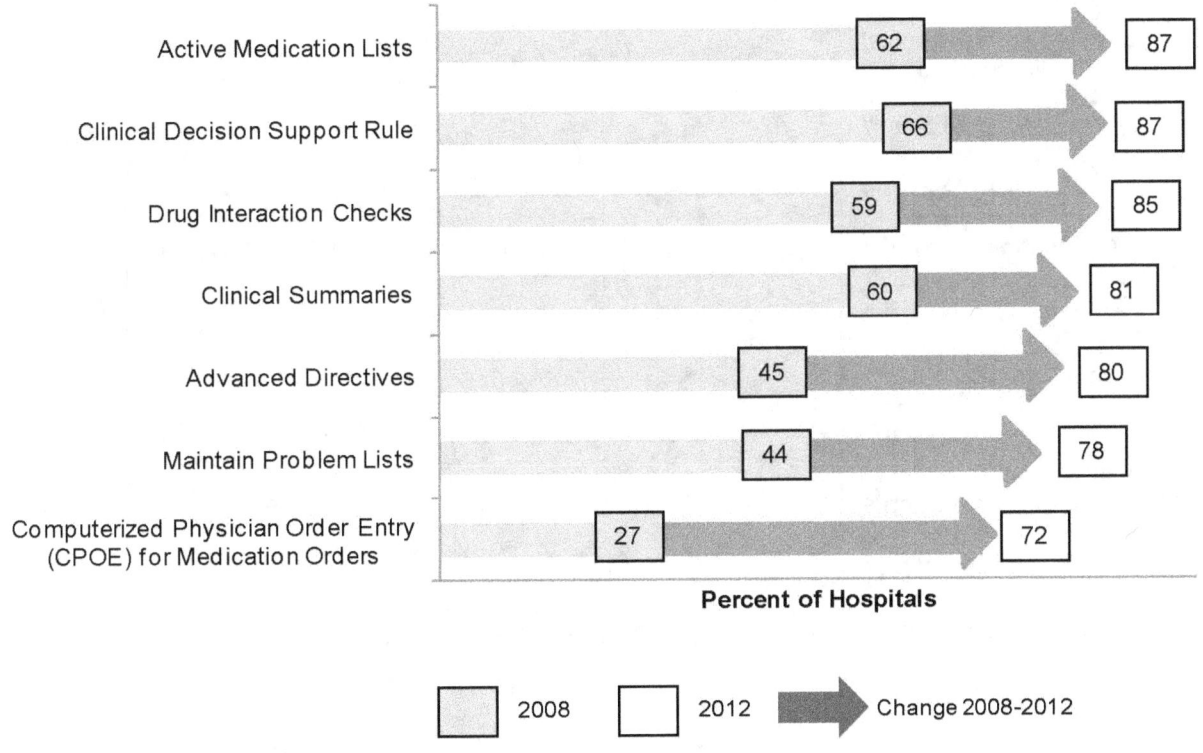

Percent of Hospitals

All differences are statistically significant from the previous year (p < 0.05).
SOURCE: ONC/AHA, AHA Annual Survey Information Technology Supplement

★ From 2008 to 2012, hospitals' capability to meet seven individual Meaningful Use objectives grew significantly, with increases ranging from 32 percent to 167 percent (Figure 4).

★ Hospital adoption of CPOE for medication orders showed the highest growth between 2008 and 2012, increasing by 167 percent.

Figure 5. Percent of physicians with computerized capabilities to meet selected EHR Incentive Programs' Meaningful Use core objectives: 2011-2012

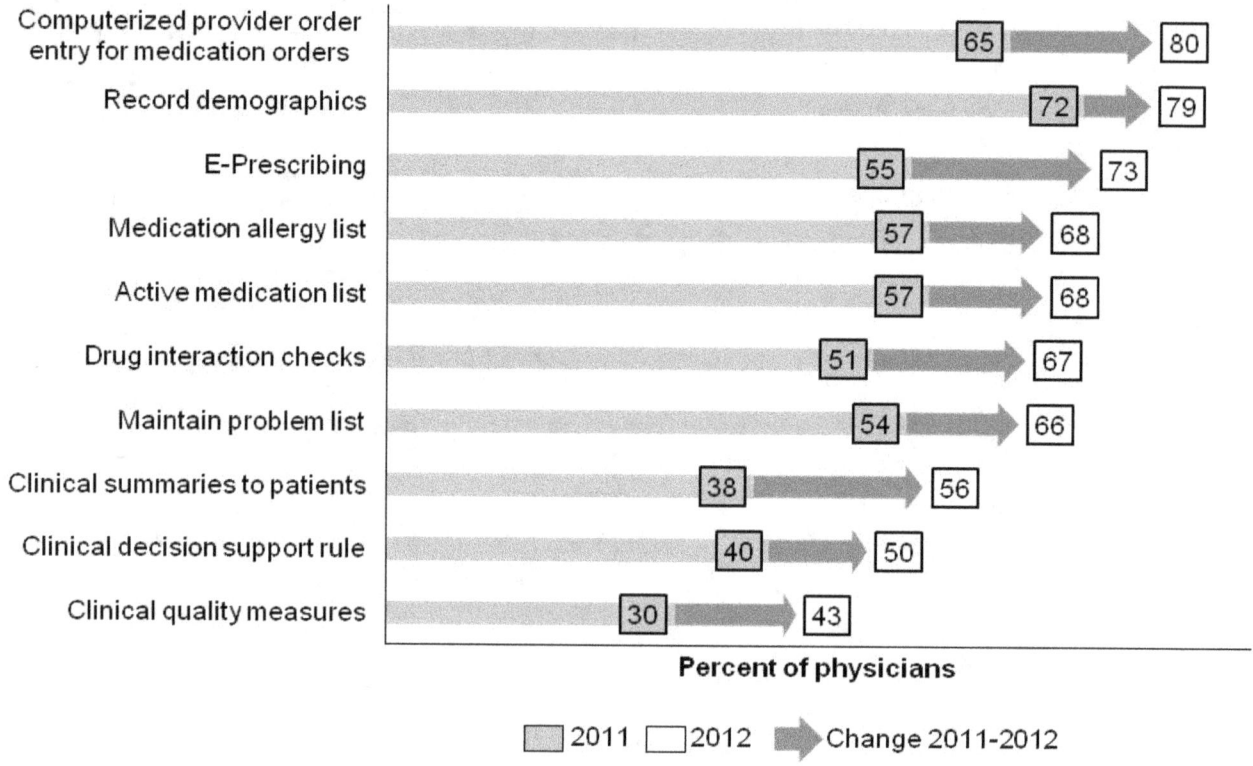

Percent of physicians

☐ 2011 ☐ 2012 ➡ Change 2011-2012

2012 is significantly different from 2011 for all computerized capabilities (p < 0.01).
SOURCE: ONC analysis of National Center for Health Statistics' 2011-2012 National Electronic Health Records Surveys.

★ Between 2011 and 2012, physician adoption of EHR technology to meet nine individual EHR Incentive Programs' Meaningful Use core objectives increased by at least 21 percent (Figure 5).

★ From 2011 to 2012, growth in physician adoption of EHR technology to engage patients and families in their health care was especially strong; the share of physicians with computerized capability to provide patients with clinical summaries after each visit increased by 46 percent.

★ Physician adoption of eight computerized capabilities to improve quality, safety, and efficiency also grew substantially, with increases ranging from 21 percent to 42 percent.

Figure 6. Percent of physicians with computerized capabilities to meet selected EHR Incentive Programs' Meaningful Use Stage 1 core objectives: 2012

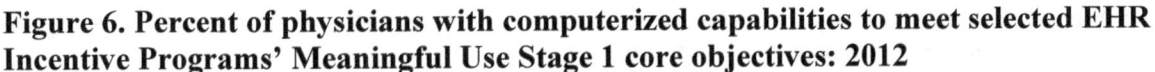

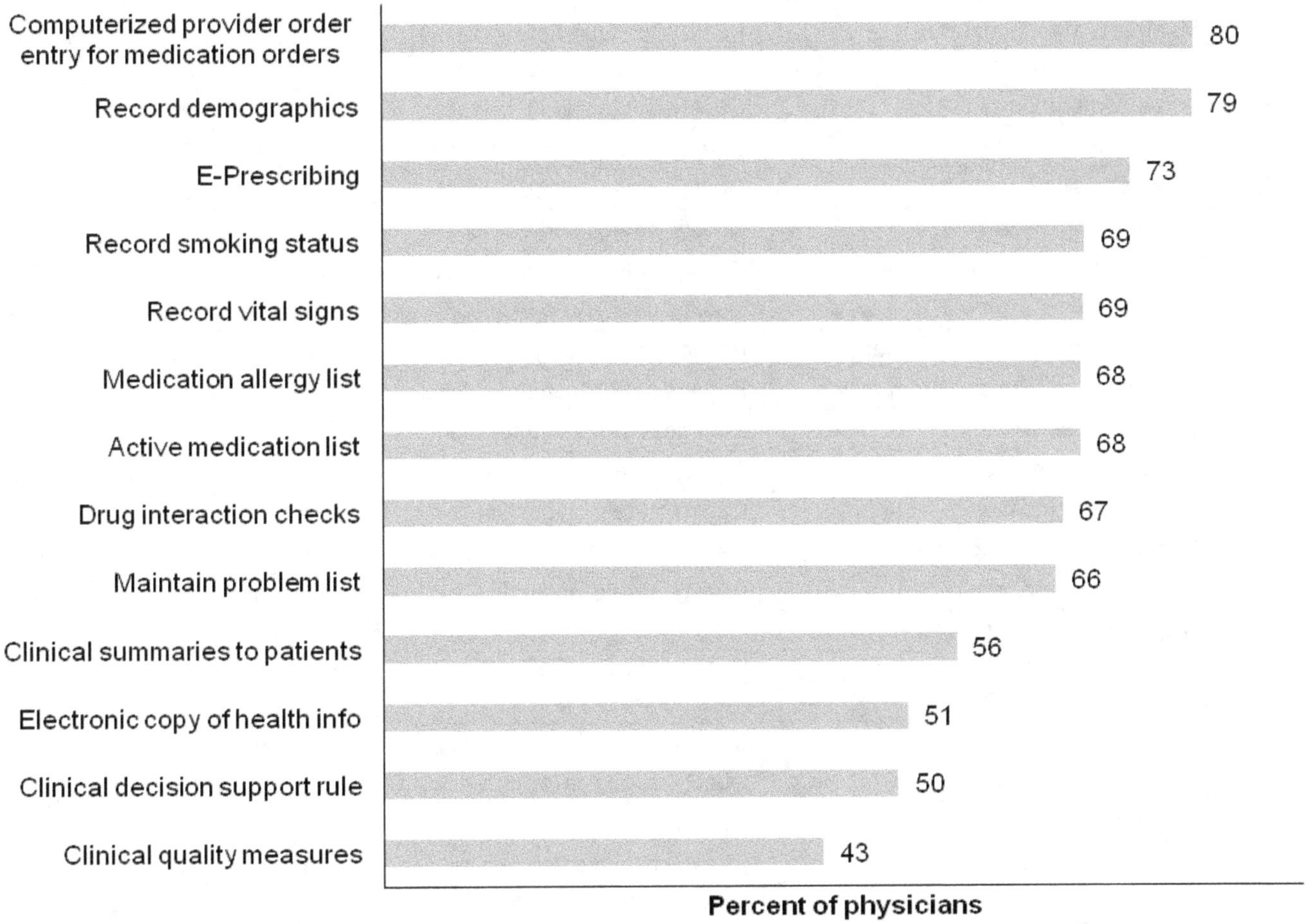

Objective	Percent
Computerized provider order entry for medication orders	80
Record demographics	79
E-Prescribing	73
Record smoking status	69
Record vital signs	69
Medication allergy list	68
Active medication list	68
Drug interaction checks	67
Maintain problem list	66
Clinical summaries to patients	56
Electronic copy of health info	51
Clinical decision support rule	50
Clinical quality measures	43

Percent of physicians

NOTE: These computerized capabilities correspond to 13 of 15 Meaningful Use core objectives for Stage 1; survey data were not available two objectives: perform a test of capacity to electronically exchange clinical information and protect electronic health information.
SOURCE: ONC analysis of the National Center for Health Statistics' 2012 National Electronic Health Records Survey.

★ In 2012, half or more of office-based physicians had adopted EHR technology to meet twelve individual EHR Incentive Programs' Meaningful Use Stage 1 core objectives (Figure 6).

★ In 2012, at least two-thirds of physicians had computerized capabilities to meet nine individual Meaningful Use core objectives to improve quality, safety, and efficiency.

Table 1. Percent of non-federal acute care hospitals with capability to meet EHR Incentive Programs' Meaningful Use objectives: 2011-2012[ii]

Stage 1 Core Measures				
Meaningful Use Measures	Health Outcome Policy Priority	2011	2012	% Change
Medication allergy lists	Quality, safety, and efficiency	80	94	18%
Record demographics	Quality, safety, and efficiency	83	93	12%
Record smoking status	Quality, safety, and efficiency	72	92	28%
Record vital signs	Quality, safety, and efficiency	76	92	21%
Active medication lists	Quality, safety, and efficiency	75	87	16%
Clinical decision support rule	Quality, safety, and efficiency	75	87	16%
Drug interaction checks	Quality, safety, and efficiency	72	85	18%
Protect electronic health information	Privacy and security	NR	82	NR
Electronic copy of health information	Engage patients and families	50	81	62%
Clinical summaries	Engage patients and families	70	81	16%
Maintain problem lists	Quality, safety, and efficiency	57	78	37%
Clinical quality measures	Quality, safety, and efficiency	47	76	62%
Clinical information exchange	Care coordination	63	72	14%
CPOE for medication orders	Quality, safety, and efficiency	51	72	41%
Stage 1 Menu Measures				
Meaningful Use Measures	Health Outcome Policy Priority	2011	2012	% Change
Medication reconciliation	Care coordination	89	93	4%
Patient lists	Quality, safety, and efficiency	70	89	27%
Clinical lab test results	Quality, safety, and efficiency	62	89	44%
Drug formulary checks	Quality, safety, and efficiency	74	85	15%
Patient-specific education	Engage patients and families	63	83	32%
Advanced directives	Quality, safety, and efficiency	67	80	19%
Transition of care summary	Care coordination	52	77	48%
Immunization registries	Public and population health	47	63	34%
Lab results to public health agencies	Public and population health	44	57	30%
Syndromic surveillance	Public and population health	41	55	34%

NR = not reported, the 2011 estimate for Protect Electronic Health Information was not reliable.
NOTE: All differences are statistically significant from the previous year (p < 0.05).
SOURCE: ONC/AHA, AHA Annual Survey Information Technology Supplement

★ Of 24 EHR Incentive Programs' Meaningful Use objectives examined, 16 objectives had adoption rates of at least 80 percent in 2012 (Table 1).

★ In 2012, hospital adoption rates for the 14 individual Meaningful Use Stage 1 core objectives ranged from 72 percent to 94 percent. Capabilities related to improving quality, safety, and efficiency had the highest adoption rates.

★ From 2011 to 2012, hospitals' capability to meet Meaningful Use objectives grew significantly; adoption rates for 13 Meaningful Use objectives each increased by at least 20 percent between 2011 and 2012.

[ii] Data is only available for 14 of the Meaningful Use core objectives.

EHR ADOPTION AMONG PROVIDERS INELIGIBLE FOR THE EHR INCENTIVE PROGRAM

Based upon the data that are currently available, which in some cases is dated, adoption of computerized technology varies among providers ineligible for the EHR Incentive Programs. A recent national survey of community-based behavioral health care providers found that approximately 65 percent use an EHR at one or more of their sites; one-fifth (21 percent) indicate they use an EHR across their sites, and 35 percent use a combination of paper/electronic across their sites.[18] A national survey of long-term facilities (which includes residential care communities, adult day service centers, home health agencies, nursing homes and hospices) was conducted in 2012 though results are not yet available.[19] Older, national surveys conducted across various types of facilities show variation in EHR adoption rates by setting. A 2010 national survey of residential care facilities found that 17 percent used any EHR, 3 percent had a basic EHR system and that more than half (55 percent) of these facilities had one or more of six electronic capabilities associated with a basic EHR.[20] Approximately 4 in 10 nursing homes (43 percent) had adopted any EHR and 2 in 10 had a basic EHR in 2004; among home and hospice care providers, 41 percent had adopted any EHR, and 10 percent had a basic EHR system in 2007.[21] A 2011 survey of long-term acute care hospitals and rehabilitation hospitals show EHR adoption rates are lower than acute care settings.[22]

E-Prescribing Activity by Physicians and Pharmacies

Recognizing the importance of e-prescribing in improving patient care, a number of programs seek to increase e-prescribing. The Medicare Improvements for Patients and Providers Act of 2008 established a voluntary CMS Electronic Prescribing (eRx) Incentive Program. The eRx program provides incentive payments for eligible Medicare providers who satisfactorily report successful e-prescribing activity from 2009 through 2013. The eRx program also adjusts the payment of eligible providers who do not become successful electronic prescribers.

In addition, under the EHR Incentive Programs, eligible professionals are required to electronically prescribe as part of Meaningful Use of certified EHR technology. E-prescribing has dramatically increased since these two programs have been implemented.[23] The percent of physicians e-prescribing using an EHR on one of the nation's largest e-prescribing network (Surescripts) increased almost eight-fold from 7 percent in December 2008 to over half of physicians (54 percent) in December 2012.[24,25] In the same period, the percent of community pharmacies active on the Surescripts network grew from 69 percent to 94 percent. The percent of new and renewal prescriptions sent electronically nationwide between 2008 and 2012 has increased ten-fold to approximately 47 percent.

Figure 7. Number of e-prescribers on the Surescripts Network and pharmacies not active on Surescripts Network

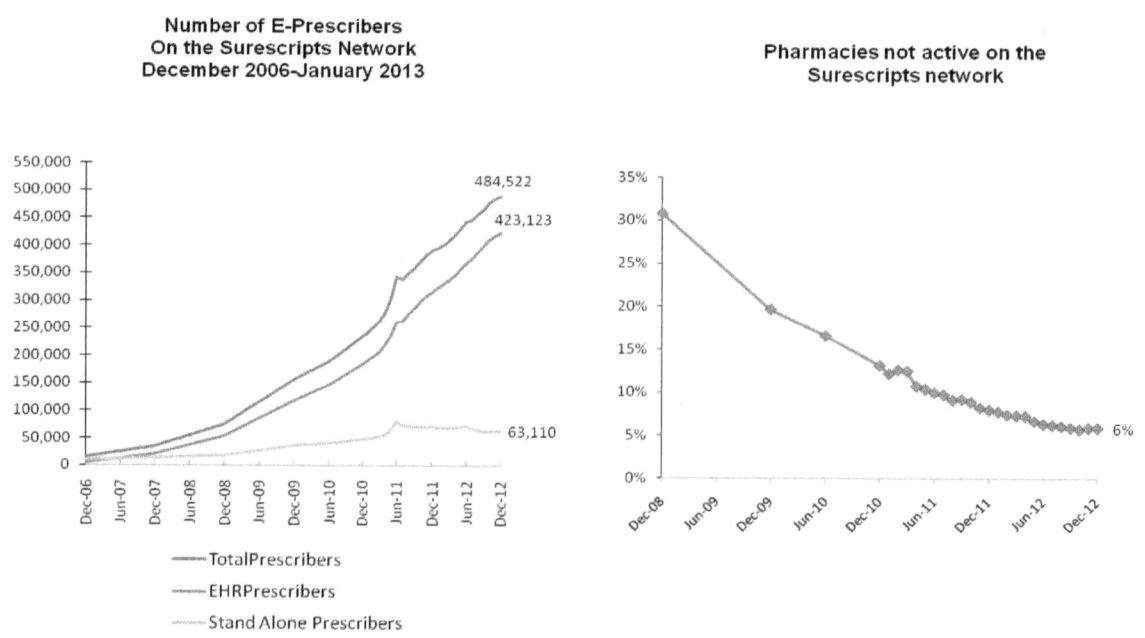

SOURCE: ONC analysis of Surescripts data.

★ Nationally, the number of providers using EHRs to e-prescribe has rapidly increased to over 400,000 as of December 2012 (Figure 7).

★ As of December 2012, very few community pharmacies nationwide (6 percent) are not actively engaged in e-prescribing on the Surescripts network.

Figure 8. Percent of physicians e-prescribing using an EHR in 2008 and 2012

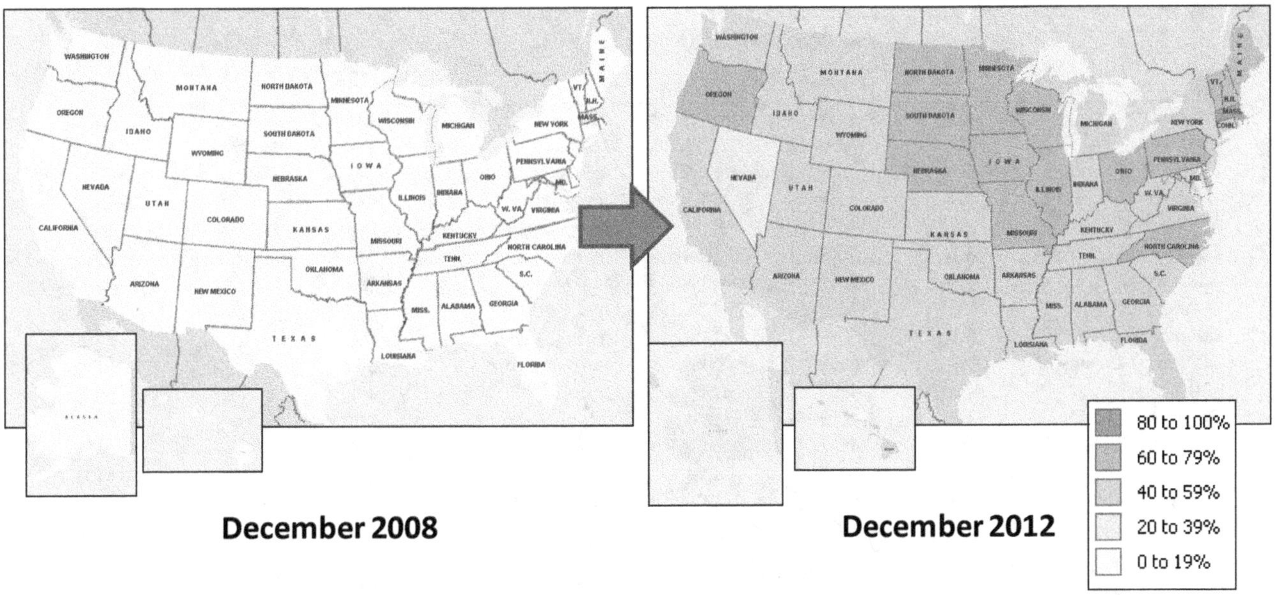

December 2008   December 2012

Legend:
- 80 to 100%
- 60 to 79%
- 40 to 59%
- 20 to 39%
- 0 to 19%

SOURCE: ONC analysis of physician prescriber data from Surescripts. Denominator from SK&A 2011 full-year file

★ The percent of physicians e-prescribing using an EHR has increased eight-fold from 7 percent in 2008 to 54 percent in 2012 (Figure 8).

★ As of December 2012, thirty-four states had more than half of their physicians e-prescribing using an EHR on the Surescripts Network.

Table 2. New and renewal prescriptions sent electronically in 2008 and 2012, by state

State	New and Renewals 2008	New and Renewals 2012	Percentage Point Increase	State	New and Renewals 2008	New and Renewals 2012	Percentage Point Increase
United States	4%	47%	43%	Missouri	4%	72%	68%
Alabama	2%	39%	37%	Montana	1%	45%	44%
Alaska	2%	33%	31%	Nebraska	2%	48%	46%
Arizona	6%	60%	54%	Nevada	9%	37%	28%
Arkansas	2%	43%	41%	New Hampshire	3%	64%	61%
California	3%	38%	35%	New Jersey	5%	34%	29%
Colorado	4%	39%	35%	New Mexico	2%	45%	43%
Connecticut	6%	46%	40%	New York	3%	43%	40%
Delaware	7%	53%	46%	North Carolina	6%	52%	46%
District of Columbia	3%	31%	28%	North Dakota	0%	57%	57%
Florida	4%	40%	36%	Ohio	4%	80%	76%
Georgia	2%	40%	38%	Oklahoma	2%	44%	42%
Hawaii	1%	45%	44%	Oregon	4%	58%	54%
Idaho	4%	44%	40%	Pennsylvania	6%	47%	41%
Illinois	4%	48%	44%	Rhode Island	17%	57%	40%
Indiana	3%	48%	45%	South Carolina	1%	42%	41%
Iowa	2%	60%	58%	South Dakota	1%	60%	59%
Kansas	3%	49%	46%	Tennessee	4%	39%	35%
Kentucky	3%	44%	41%	Texas	3%	44%	41%
Louisiana	3%	32%	29%	Utah	1%	41%	40%
Maine	6%	60%	54%	Vermont	4%	61%	57%
Maryland	5%	42%	37%	Virginia	3%	46%	43%
Massachusetts	20%	67%	47%	Washington	4%	54%	50%
Michigan	8%	49%	41%	West Virginia	3%	35%	32%
Minnesota	4%	80%	76%	Wisconsin	2%	65%	63%
Mississippi	1%	39%	38%	Wyoming	2%	39%	37%

SOURCE: ONC analysis of Surescripts data

★ There has been more than a ten-fold increase in the percent of new and renewal prescriptions sent electronically nationwide between 2008 and 2012 (Table 2).

★ In 2012, states' rates of sending new prescriptions and renewals prescriptions electronically ranged from 31 percent to 80 percent.

★ From 2008 to 2012, thirteen states' rates of sending new prescriptions and renewals electronically increased by 50 percentage points or more.

Figure 9. Percent of new and renewal prescriptions sent electronically in 2012, by state

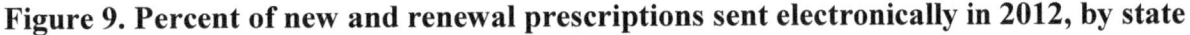

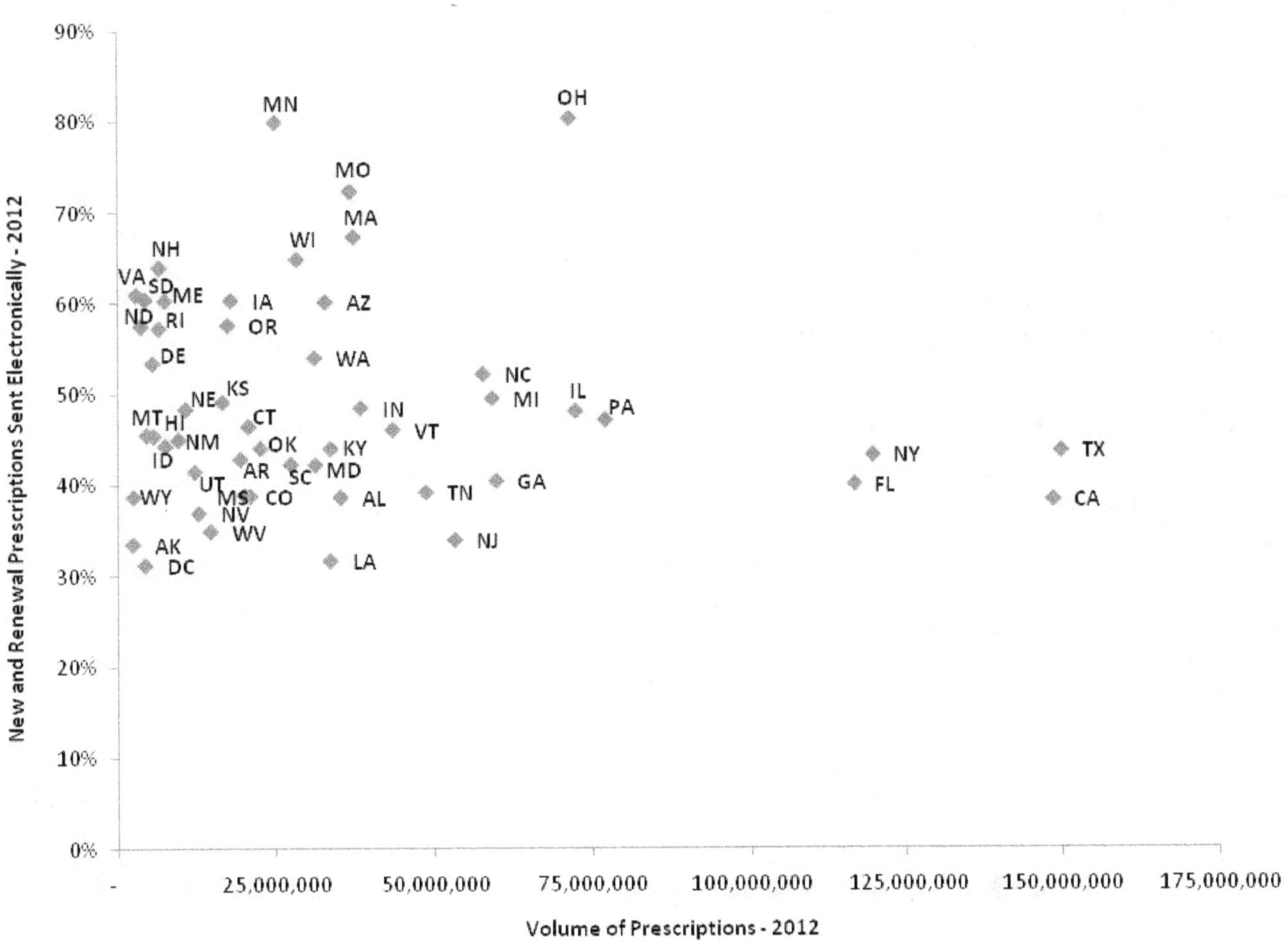

Note: 1,746,471,461 new and renewal prescriptions sent electronically in 2012 nationally.
SOURCE: ONC analysis of annual prescription data from Surescripts, 2012.

★ In 2012, all states have at least 30 percent of new and renewal prescriptions transmitted electronically (Figure 9).

★ In seventeen states, over half of all new and renewal prescriptions are now sent electronically.

PROGRAMS THAT ENABLE HEALTH IT ADOPTION

THE MEDICARE AND MEDICAID EHR INCENTIVE PROGRAMS: PROGRESS TOWARDS MEANINGFUL USE OF EHRS

The CMS Medicare and Medicaid EHR Incentive Programs provide financial incentives for the "Meaningful Use" of certified EHR technology. In addition to the incentives, providers who fail to demonstrate meaningful use will be subject to payment adjustments under Medicare beginning in 2015. CMS has established, through notice and comment rulemaking, objectives for Meaningful Use that eligible professionals, eligible hospitals, and Critical Access Hospitals must meet in order to receive an incentive payment.[26] The share of providers that have been paid under this program has grown significantly and is spread across the U.S. (Figure 10 and 11).

Figure 10. Progress of eligible providers in CMS EHR Incentive Programs: April 2013

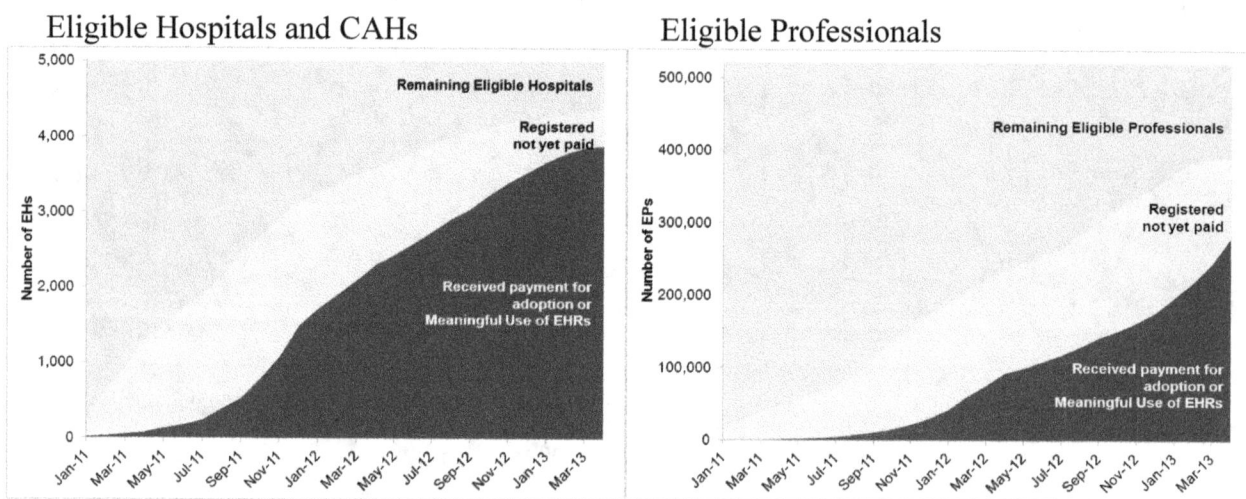

SOURCE: CMS EHR Incentive Program data

★ As of April 2013, over 394,000 of the nation's eligible professionals and hospitals have registered in the Medicare and Medicaid systems with an intent to participate in the EHR Incentive Programs.

★ As of April 2013, more than 291,000 professionals, representing more than half of the nation's eligible professionals, have received incentive payments through the EHR Incentive Programs. Over 3,800 hospitals, representing about 80 percent of eligible hospitals, which includes Critical Access Hospitals, have received incentive payments through this program as well.

Figure 11. Share of physicians, nurse practitioners, and physician assistants paid under the Medicare and Medicaid EHR Incentive Programs

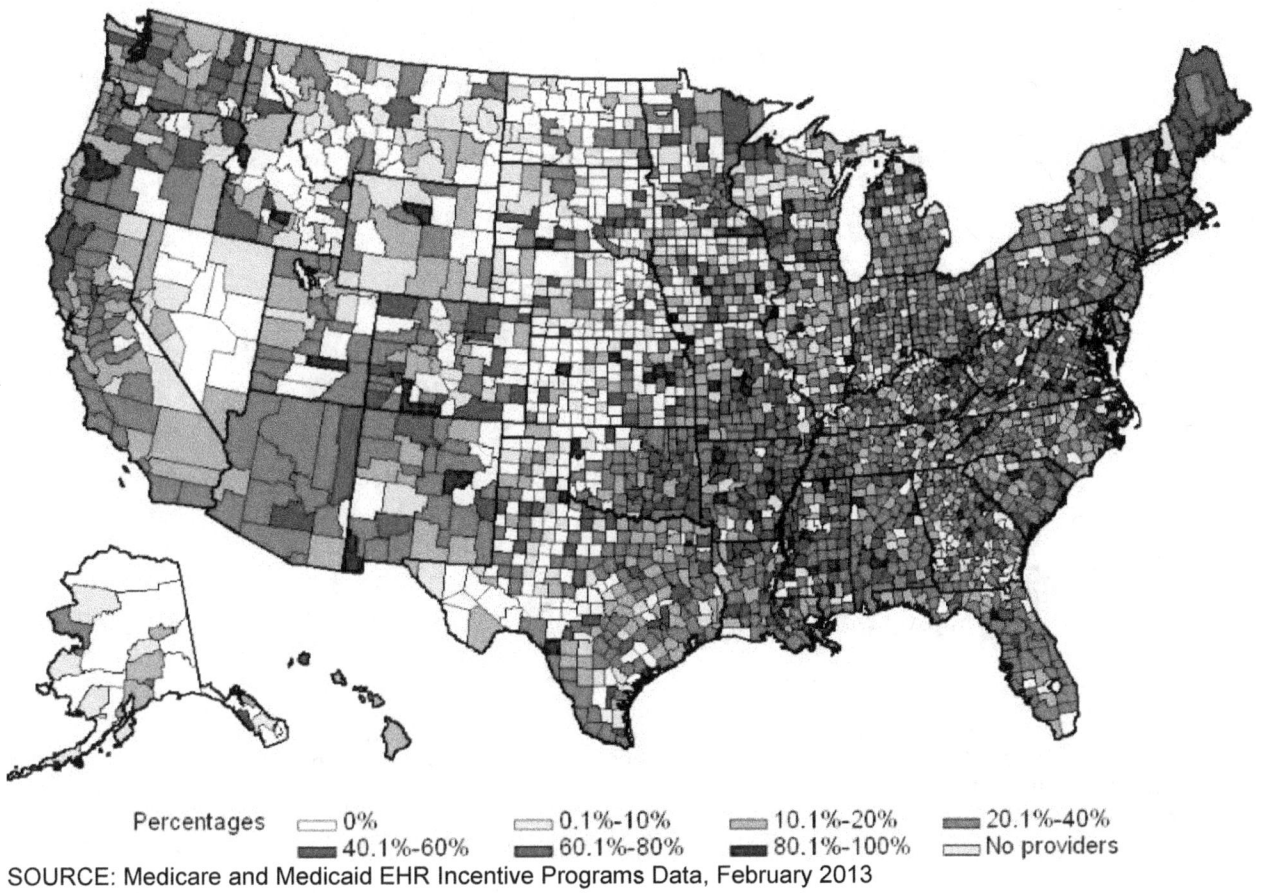

Percentages
- ☐ 0%
- ☐ 0.1%-10%
- ☐ 10.1%-20%
- ☐ 20.1%-40%
- ☐ 40.1%-60%
- ☐ 60.1%-80%
- ☐ 80.1%-100%
- ☐ No providers

SOURCE: Medicare and Medicaid EHR Incentive Programs Data, February 2013

Table 3. Medicare and Medicaid EHR Incentive Programs participation among eligible professionals as of April 2013

	Total		Non-Metropolitan Areas		Metropolitan Areas	
Number of Eligible Professionals Registered (thousands)						
	N	%	N	%	N	%
Total	390.5	100%	45.7	12%	344.8	88%
Medicaid	127.0	100%	19.1	15%	107.9	85%
Medicare	263.4	100%	26.7	10%	236.7	90%
Number of Eligible Professionals Receiving Payment (thousands)						
Total	291.3	100%	34.1	12%	257.2	88%
Medicaid	88.9	100%	14.1	16%	74.8	84%
Medicare	202.4	100%	20.1	10%	182.3	90%
Total Estimated Ambulatory Physicians, Nurse Practitioners, and Physician Assistants*	716.1	100%	82.6	12%	633.5	88%

NOTES: This estimate includes all physicians, NPs, and PAs, not all of whom are eligible for the incentive programs. There were an estimated 521.6 thousand eligible professionals in 2011. Estimates of eligible professionals by metropolitan status are not available.

Non-metropolitan are defined as counties that are outside of a Metropolitan Statistical Area. Primary care Health Professional Shortage Areas (HPSAs) are defined as zip codes considered by CMS to be eligible for primary care HPSA bonus payment (http://www.cms.gov/Medicare/Medicare-Fee-for-Service-Payment/HPSAPSAPhysicianBonuses/index.html). Total eligible professionals estimate is from the Final Rule for Stage 1 of the Medicare and Medicaid EHR Incentive Programs. Information on total ambulatory physicians, nurse practitioners, and physicians' assistants is derived from SK&A Information Services Office-Based Provider Database, 2011

★ As of April 2013, the distribution of eligible professionals registered or paid by the Medicare and Medicaid EHR Incentive Program was similar regardless of metropolitan status (Table 3).

★ Overall, twelve percent of ambulatory care providers were located in non-metropolitan or rural areas; similarly, 12 percent of eligible professionals that registered for or received payment from the EHR Incentive Program were located in rural areas.

Table 4. Medicare and Medicaid EHR Incentive Programs participation among eligible hospitals and critical access hospitals as of April 2013

Hospital Type	Number (Percent) of Hospitals, in Hundreds			
	Registered with either Medicare or Medicaid Incentive Program	Attested to Meaningful Use	Received payment for adopting certified EHR or attesting to Meaningful Use	Total hospitals
Total	43.7 (88%)	30.1 (60%)	38.8 (78%)	49.8
Critical Access Hospitals[iii]	11.2 (84%)	7.5 (56%)	9.1 (68%)	13.3
Hospitals (not including Critical Access Hospitals)				
In non-metropolitan areas	9.0 (95%)	6.5 (68%)	8.3 (87%)	9.5
In metropolitan areas	23.5 (87%)	16.1 (60%)	21.3 (79%)	27.0

NOTES: Estimates of total hospitals reflect the number of hospitals certified by the Centers for Medicare & Medicaid Services as of June 2012 with hospital sub-types of short term, children's, or Critical Access Hospital. Non-metropolitan areas defined as counties that are outside of a Metropolitan Statistical Area. All counts are unduplicated. Hospitals receiving payment for adopting certified EHR or attesting to Meaningful Use includes hospitals that have received payment from either the Medicare or Medicaid EHR Incentive Programs.

★ Eighty-four percent of CAHs in the nation have registered for EHR incentive payments and more than two-thirds (sixty-eight percent) of CAHs had received incentive payments for adopting certified EHRs or attesting to Meaningful Use as of April 2013 (Table 4).

★ Critical Access Hospitals' registration and payment rates are similar to the overall percentage of hospitals that have registered (84 percent vs. 88 percent), but slightly lower in the overall percentage that received payment (68 percent vs. 78 percent). RECs are providing technical assistance and education to three out of every four CAHs to enable these hospitals to demonstrate Meaningful Use of EHRs.

★ Among hospitals that are not CAHs, a slightly higher percentage of the facilities that are located in non-metropolitan areas have registered and received payment (95 percent registered and 87 percent paid), compared with hospitals located in metropolitan areas (87 percent registered, 79 percent paid).

[iii] *Critical access hospital*: A facility that is Medicare-certified to receive cost-based reimbursement. Generally, to qualify as a CAH, it must be at least 35 miles (or 15 miles in mountainous terrain or areas with only secondary roads) from the nearest hospital or CAH, have a maximum of 25 inpatient beds, and maintain an annual average length of stay of 96 hours or less for their acute care patients. http://www.flexmonitoring.org/cahlistRA.cgi

ALIGNING BOTH HEALTH IT AND ELECTRONIC STANDARDS PROGRAMS

As the nation's largest healthcare payer, CMS operationalized the Medicare and Medicaid EHR Incentive Program by creating program policies and supporting systems necessary for its implementation. Through the EHR Incentive Programs, CMS developed program requirements through notice and comment rulemaking, which include the Meaningful Use objectives. These are measures and thresholds that eligible professionals, eligible hospitals, and CAHs must meet in order to receive an incentive payment. CMS also created the necessary program infrastructure in order to successfully implement the EHR Incentive Programs in accordance with existing payment policies, program eligibility criteria, as well as creating the interface with external systems. Below is an overview of the CMS efforts to increase adoption of health information technology and health information exchange.

Office of eHealth Standards and Services (OESS)

OESS administers the Medicare and Medicaid EHR Incentive Programs, is the agency lead for privacy policy and compliance, and coordinates CMS' efforts to share healthcare data freely and easily among patients, physicians, healthcare providers, and health plans to improve health outcomes and reduce costs. Some of the health reform initiatives to improve interoperability include the standardization of operating rules and electronic transactions for healthcare billing and payment and preparation for the transition to using the ICD-10 code sets for improved capture of granular health care information for both billing and quality measurement reporting.

Office of Information Systems (OIS)

OIS provides information technology and program management support for the EHR Incentive Programs. OIS, in coordination with OESS, designed, developed, and maintains the National Level Repository (NLR) of EHR data, Registration and Attestation (RNA), as well as the HITECH Research & Support User Interface (R&S UI) systems. OIS also coordinates and monitors numerous interfaces between CMS systems and other entities ensuring successful data transmission. OIS manages and oversees the EHR Information Center, which responds to provider inquiries about the program, manages system operations support, and oversees data quality and reporting.

Office of Financial Management (OFM)

OFM determines provider eligibility for participation in the EHR Incentive Programs, generates and distributes the incentive payments, and conducts pre- and post-payment audits to assure program integrity.

Centers for Medicaid and CHIP Services (CMCS)

The Medicaid EHR Incentive Program eligibility and program policies are determined by CMCS in coordination with each state. CMCS plays a leadership role in the coordination within and among states to support the implementation of EHRs, and coordinates with state Medicaid program expansion and health marketplace efforts.

Centers for Clinical Quality and Standards (CCSQ)

CCSQ seeks to improve quality of care through the use of robust CQMs (Clinical Quality Measures), timely feedback to hospitals and physicians, and Meaningful Use of EHRs. The next phase of the EHR Incentive Programs will encourage the adoption of broad scale electronic reporting of quality data. CCSQ is working to minimize provider burden by implementing a unified set of electronic clinical quality measures (eCQMs) and electronic reporting requirements. CMS has worked with partners and representatives from industry to identify and finalize a set of unified quality measures that eligible health care providers could report to satisfy some of the various requirements of multiple programs, such as the Physician Quality Reporting System (PQRS) and Physician Value-Based Modifier, in addition to the EHR Incentive Programs requirements for clinical quality measure reporting. CCSQ is also taking measures such as the following to minimize provider reporting burden:

- Enabling synchronized performance and submission reporting periods
- Allowing participating providers to make one submission of electronic CQM (eCQM) data for multiple programs
- Using the same CQMs and electronic specifications across programs
- Maximizing efficiency by using eCQM data submitted by providers for multiple quality programs

CCSQ quality reporting programs include the e-Prescribing Incentive program (which was described earlier in the adoption section of this report), the PQRS reporting program and the Hospital IQR Program. The PQRS is a reporting program that uses a combination of incentive payments and payment adjustments to promote reporting of quality information by eligible professionals. The Hospital IQR Program provides a financial incentive to hospitals the successfully report designated quality measures to CMS and provides CMS with data to help consumers make more informed decisions about their health care. CMS is aligning the Hospital IQR with the EHR Incentive Programs to allow hospitals to submit unified measures through a single submission method.

Center for Medicare and Medicaid Innovation (Innovation Center)

The Innovation Center identifies, creates, tests, and evaluates new payment and service delivery models to reduce program expenditures while preserving or enhancing the quality of care furnished to Medicare, Medicaid, and CHIP beneficiaries. One model that relies heavily on health IT is the Pioneer Accountable Care Organization (ACO) model, which is comprised of groups of doctors, hospitals, and other health care providers who come together voluntarily to provide coordinated high quality care to the Medicare patients they serve. Interoperable Health IT systems allow these providers to coordinate care across providers and settings and ensuring that patients, especially the chronically ill, get the right care at the right time, avoiding unnecessary duplication of services and preventing medical errors. When a Pioneer ACO succeeds in both delivering high-quality care and spending health care dollars more wisely, it will share in the savings it achieves for the Medicare program. Health IT enables implementation of these new payment and delivery models by facilitating data exchange and data analytics necessary for Pioneer ACOs, bundled payments, patient-centered medical homes, and other efforts.

ONC's Health IT Regional Extension Centers Program: Helping Primary Care Providers Achieve Milestones related to EHR Adoption & Meaningful Use

ONC's Regional Extension Center (REC) program consists of 62 heterogeneous non-profit organizations and a national Health Information Technology Research Center (HITRC) that provides state-of-the-art technical assistance on best practices for EHR adoption. RECs have directly assisted providers in their understanding of the EHR Incentive Programs, supported providers during the EHR selection process; and, trained practice staff in workflow redesign, project management, and technology and security assessments. Additionally, RECs have supported many provider practices with ongoing training and optimization of their workflow to achieve Meaningful Use of their certified EHR technology.

Figure 12. Number of REC assisted providers by EHR implementation milestone

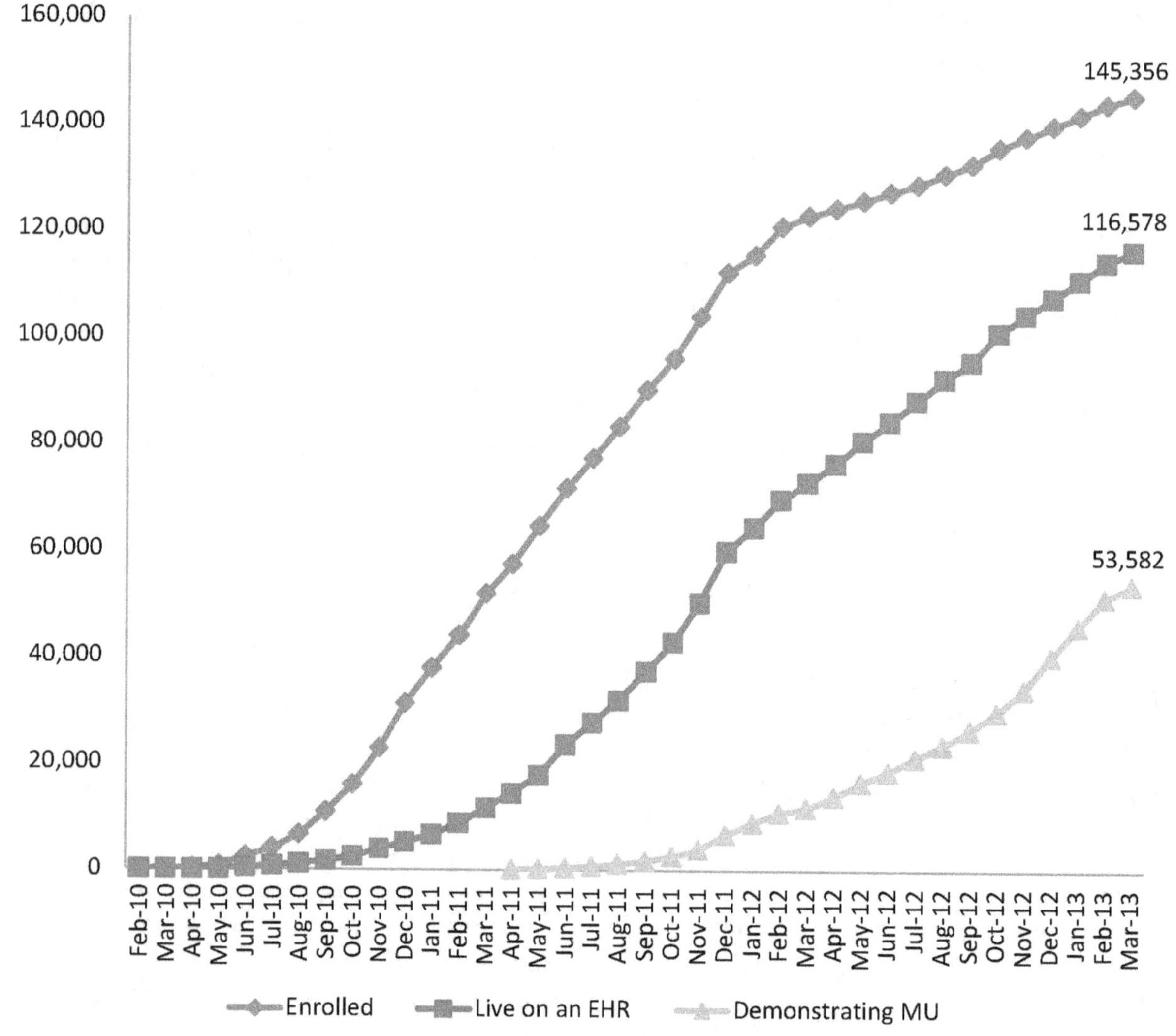

SOURCE: ONC Customer Relationship Management (CRM) Database, Data as of March, 2013

The REC program has been successfully assisting primary care providers nationwide to adopt EHRs and demonstrate Meaningful Use. The key REC milestones include providers opting to participate in the REC Program (Figure 13), participating providers going live on an EHR system, and these providers achieving Meaningful Use of certified EHR technology. The REC Program surpassed the 2012 HHS High Priority Goal of providing assistance to 100,000 primary care providers (Figure 12). A Government Accountability Office (GAO) report found that Medicare providers working with RECs were over 2.3 times more likely to receive an EHR incentive payment then those who were not working with a REC.[27] Almost half (46 percent) of providers that received incentives from the Medicaid EHR Incentive Program for attesting to Meaningful Use, and one-fifth (21 percent) of providers that received incentives from the Medicare EHR Incentive Program have participated in the REC program.

Figure 13. Percent of primary care providers participating with an REC

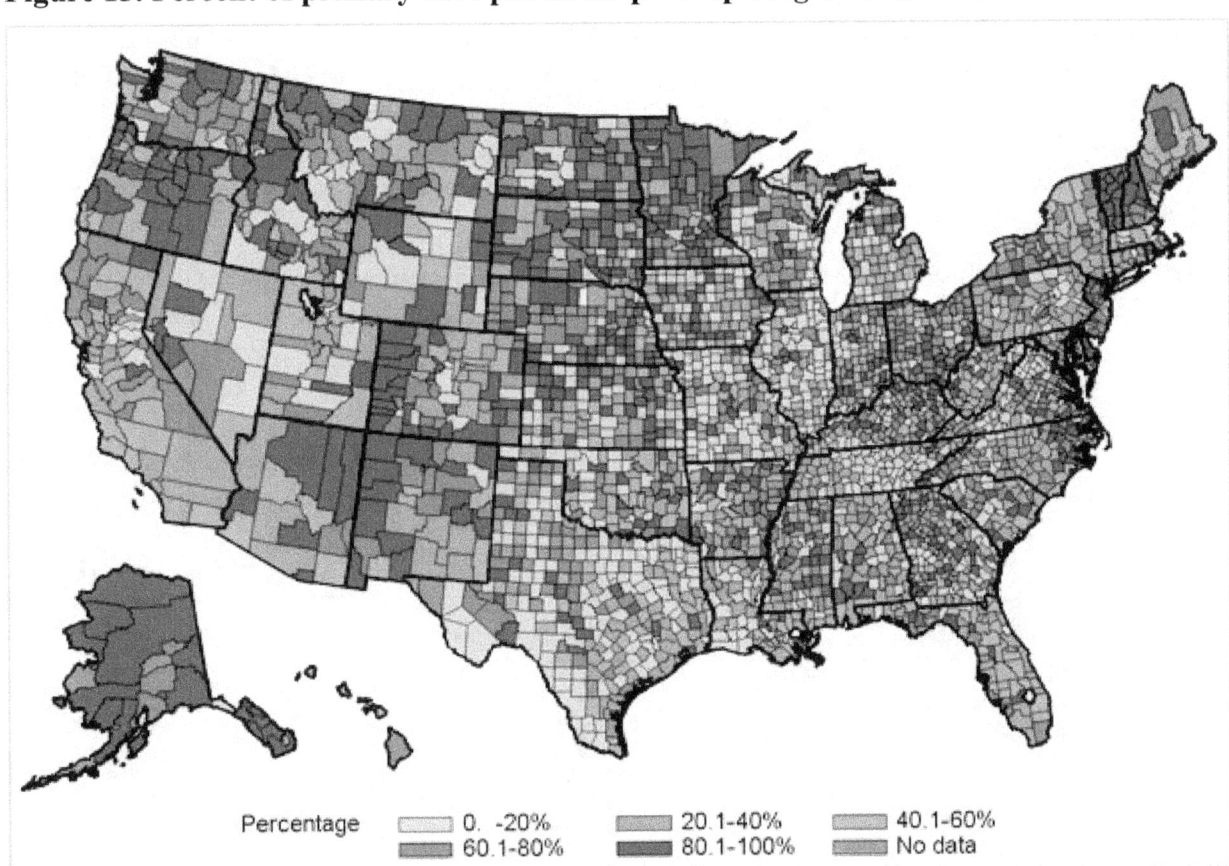

SOURCE: ONC Customer Relationship Management (CRM) Database, February 2013

Table 5. Primary care providers participating with RECs by type

Degree	Total PCPs Nationwide	# of PCPs Enrolled	% of Total Enrolled PCPs	Proportion of PCPs Enrolled with RECs	# of PCPs Demonstrating MU	Proportion of REC PCPs Demonstrating MU
MD/DO	238,352	101,640	76%	43%	43,254	43%
NP	41,746	20,306	15%	49%	4,777	24%
PA	22,628	9,654	7%	43%	2,372	25%
CNMW	NA	2,006	2%	NA	392	20%
TOTAL	302,726	133,606	100%	44%	50,795	38%

SOURCE: ONC Customer Relationship Management (CRM) Database, maintained by the Office of Provider Adoption and Support (OPAS) at ONC, data as of March, 26th 2013. Provider denominators obtained from the SK&A Office-based Providers Database, Q4, 2011.

★ RECs have worked with over 133,000 primary care providers in nearly 30,000 different practices, representing approximately 43 percent of all the primary care physicians and 49 percent of all nurse practitioners nationwide (Table 5).

★ As part of their long-term business sustainability strategy, the RECs are also working with over 10,000 specialists who have asked for assistance in achieving Meaningful Use.

The RECs are successfully reaching out to support primary care providers operating in medically underserved regions nationwide to implement certified EHR technology and demonstrate Meaningful Use. Based upon a recent study, REC enrollment rates were highest in rural areas.[28] Specifically, REC enrollment rates were found to be higher for small rural (non-CBSA, 56 percent) and micropolitan areas (47 percent) compared to urban or metropolitan areas (Table 6).

REC enrollment rates were also found to be highest in counties with the greatest health professional shortages, in particular for whole-county HPSAs, which are areas that have shortages spanning entire county area and population (52 percent) and geographic HPSAs, which have shortages in specific geographic areas within the county but not the entire county (42 percent).

Table 6. REC Enrollment Nationwide by Rural and Provider Shortage Area Designations

	% Enrolled with REC
Rural Designation	
Overall	40%
Metropolitan	38%
Micropolitan (large rural)	47%
Non-CBSA (small rural)	56%
Healthcare Provider Shortage Area (HPSA) Designation	
Non-HPSA	40%
Geographic HPSA	42%
Population Group HPSA	39%
Whole County HPSA	52%

NOTES: CBSA indicates Core Based Statistical Area. HPSA indicates Health Professional Shortage Area. Designations taken from the 2010 Area Resource File. Under this designation, counties belong to one of three categories: metropolitan (urban); micropolitan (large rural); and non-CBSA (small rural). Among these categories, non-CBSA indicates the greatest degree of rurality. County-level HPSA designations were derived from HRSA's November 2011 Primary Care HPSA data file. Counties were categorized into four categories: *non-HPSA* (no shortage); *geographic area HPSA* (shortages in specific geographic areas within the county but the not the entire county); *population group HPSA* (shortages for specific population groups that may be present in a specific geographic area with the county or across the entire count); and *whole-county HPSA* (shortages spanning entire county area and population). Among these categories, whole-county HPSA indicates the greatest degree of health professional shortage for a given area.
SOURCE: Analysis of REC-enrolled PCPs from ONC Customer Relationship Management (CRM) Database; Total PCPs from SK&A; as of February, 2012
Table adapted from: Samuel CA, King J, Adetosoye F, Samy L, Furukawa MF. Engaging providers in underserved areas to adopt electronic health records. *American Journal of Managed Care.* 2013;19(3):229-34.

In addition to addressing disparities in EHR adoption among providers working in underserved areas with few health professionals and rural areas, RECs have been successfully engaging primary care providers working in settings that serve medically underserved populations.[29,30] These providers historically have had lower rates of EHR adoption due to limited access to capital, staff expertise, or other technical resources. The types of settings RECs have been working with include: small group practices of 10 or fewer professionals; public hospitals; critical access hospitals; health centers; rural health clinics; and other settings that predominantly serve medically underserved populations (Table 7). Data in Table 7 show the different types of practices participating with the REC program, including whether they demonstrated meaningful use as measured by ONC milestones. Note that this does not necessarily indicate receipt of an incentive payment under the Medicare and Medicaid EHR Incentive Programs.

Table 7. The type of practices participating with an REC

Practice Type*	# of Providers Enrolled with RECs	% of Total REC-Enrolled Providers	# of Providers Demonstrating MU through ONC Milestones	Proportion of REC Providers who are demonstrating MU	# of Practices	Avg # of Providers per Practice
Private Practice 1 - 10	51,903	36%	21,797	42%	23,611	2
Specialty Practice	3,019	2%	807	27%	603	5
Rural Health Clinic	3,669	3%	1,019	28%	828	4
Critical Access Hospitals	4,492	3%	992	22%	630	7
Private Practice 11+	667	0%	161	24%	49	14
Other Underserved Setting	17,578	12%	6,679	38%	1,264	14
Rural Hospital	2,418	2%	760	31%	150	16
Health Center	22,778	16%	4,853	21%	1,431	16
Practice Consortiums	21,417	15%	10,800	50%	919	24
Public Hospitals	17,415	12%	5,714	33%	465	36
TOTAL	**145,356**	**100%**	**53,582**	**37%**	**29,950**	**14**

SOURCE: ONC Customer Relationship Management (CRM) Database, maintained by the Office of Provider Adoption and Support (OPAS) at ONC, data as of March, 2013

★ The largest group of providers that RECs are assisting work in small physician practices; to date, over one-third (36 percent) of REC providers are in small practices and (42 percent) of these providers are demonstrating Meaningful Use.

★ Providers working in health centers (16 percent), practice consortiums (15 percent), and public hospitals (12 percent) also represent a large proportion of REC participants. Most health centers took advantage of the Medicaid incentive payment in year one and therefore did not need to demonstrate Meaningful Use in the first year.

Figure 14. Location of critical access and other small rural hospitals enrolled with a REC

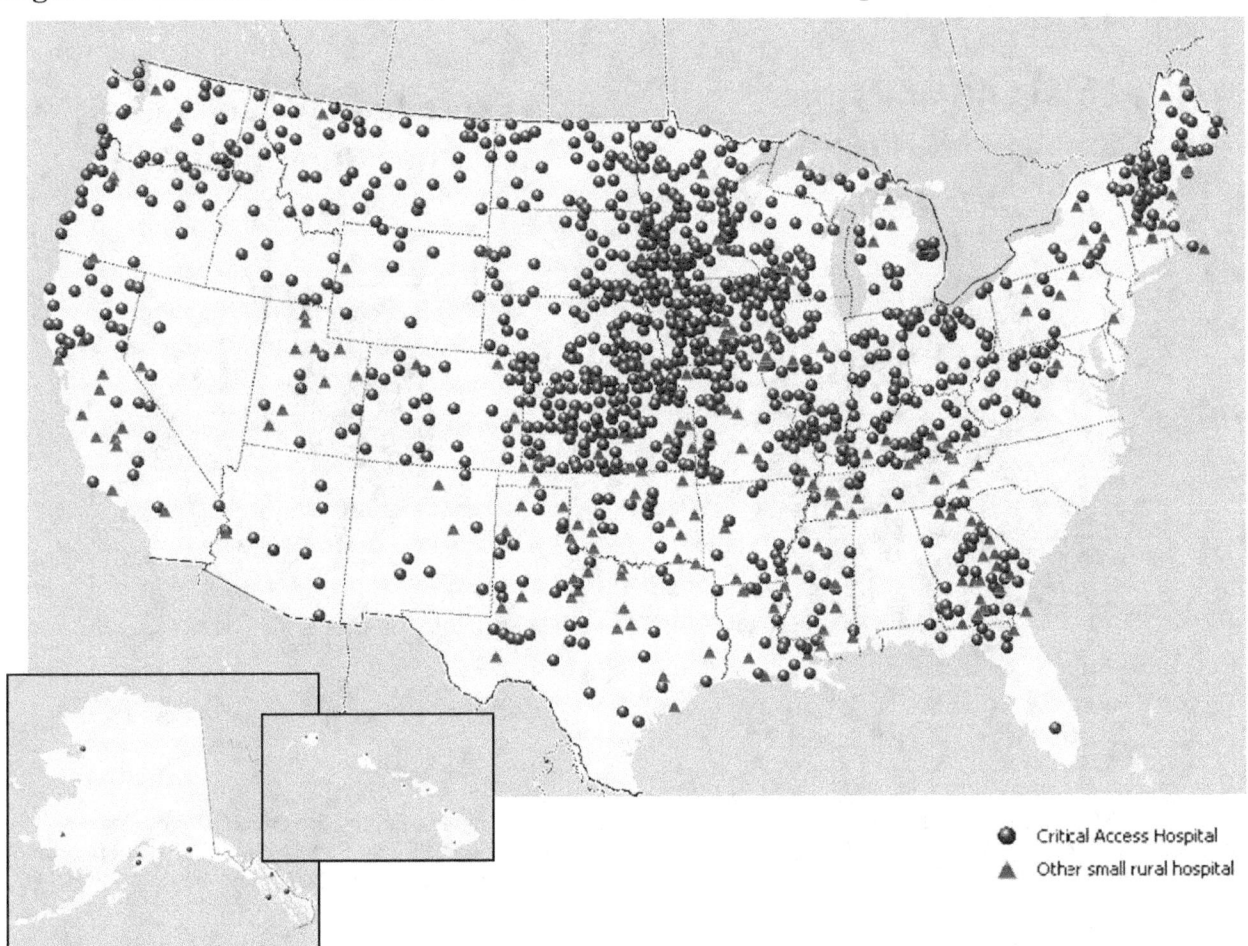

Legend:
● Critical Access Hospital
▲ Other small rural hospital

SOURCE: ONC Customer Relationship Management (CRM) Database, maintained by the Office of Provider Adoption and Support (OPAS) at ONC, a national CAH database maintained by The Flex Monitoring Team, and the Small Hospital Improvement Program (SHIP) maintained by Health Resources and Services Administration (HRSA). Data as of February 18, 2013.
Figure from: Heisey-Grove D, Hufstader M, Hollin I, Samy L, Shanks, K. Progress towards the meaningful use of electronic health records among critical access and small rural hospitals working with Regional Extension Centers. ONC Data Brief, no. 5. Washington, DC: Office of the National Coordinator for Health Information Technology, November 2012.

★ More than three-quarters (77 percent) of critical access hospitals are working with a REC.

★ Almost half (46 percent) of other small rural hospitals are working with a REC.

Figure 15. Percent of the enrolled critical access and other small rural hospitals (n=1,205) by milestone achievement

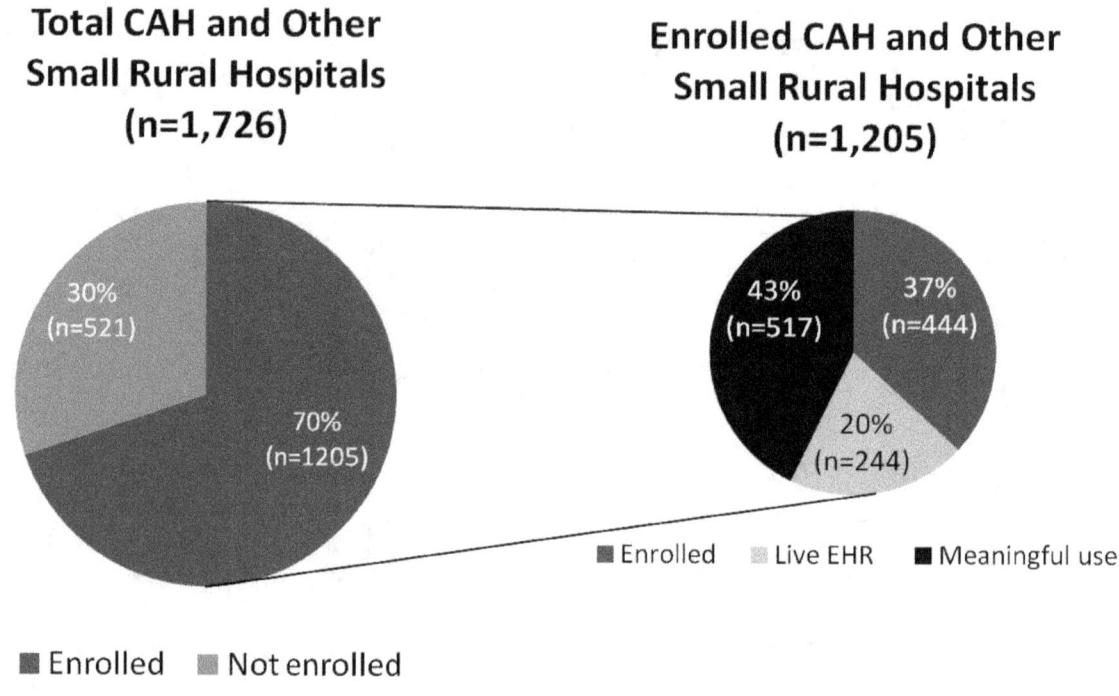

SOURCE: ONC Customer Relationship Management (CRM) Database, maintained by the Office of Provider Adoption and Support (OPAS) at ONC, a national CAH database maintained by The Flex Monitoring Team, and the Small Hospital Improvement Program (SHIP) maintained by Health Resources and Services Administration (HRSA). Data as of February 18, 2013.

★ 70 percent (1205 of 1,726) of critical access and other small rural hospitals are enrolled with a REC.

★ 63 percent (761 of 1,205) of the critical access and other small rural hospitals enrolled with a REC are using an EHR.

★ Of those critical access and other small rural hospitals that participate with a REC and are live on an EHR, 517 (68 percent) have demonstrated Meaningful Use of certified EHR technology.

Figure 16. Percent of health centers partnering with RECs by state

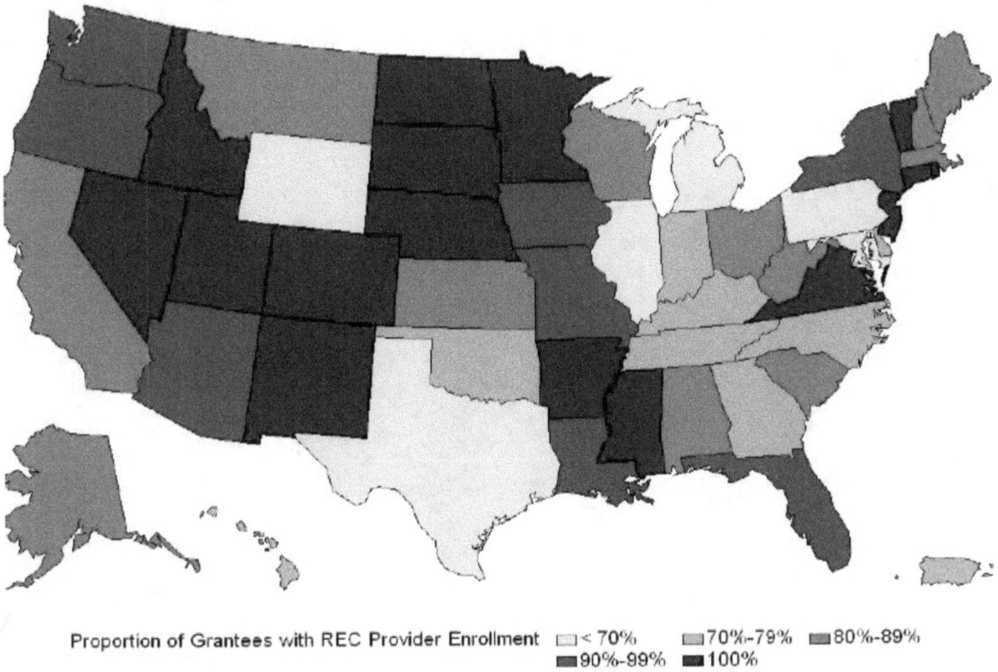

Proportion of Grantees with REC Provider Enrollment ☐ < 70%   ▨ 70%-79%   ▨ 80%-89%   ▨ 90%-99%   ▨ 100%

SOURCE: Customer ONC Customer Relationship Management (CRM) Database, maintained by the Office of Provider Adoption and Support (OPAS) at ONC, and Health Center Sites list maintained by Health Resources Services Administration (HRSA). Data as of November 25, 2012.[31]

★ A high proportion of health centers nationwide are participating with a REC (Figure 16). Over eight in ten (83 percent) health centers[iv] that serve medically underserved communities have providers enrolled with a REC.

[iv] The term "health center" is used to refer to organizations that receive grants under the Health Center Program as authorized under section 330 of the Public Health Service Act, as amended (referred to as "grantees") and FQHC Look-Alike organizations, which meet all the Health Center Program requirements but do not receive Health Center Program grants. It does not refer to FQHCs that are sponsored by tribal or Urban Indian Health Organizations, except for those that receive Health Center Program grants. In this document, unless otherwise noted, the term "health center" is used to refer to organizations that receive grants under the Health Center Program as authorized under section 330 of the Public Health Service Act, as amended (referred to as "grantees") and FQHC Look-Alike organizations, which meet all the Health Center Program requirements but do not receive Health Center Program grants. It does not refer to FQHCs that are sponsored by tribal or Urban Indian Health Organizations, except for those that receive Health Center Program grants.

Figure 17. Cumulative amount of CMS EHR incentive funds received by eligible professionals in REC-Enrolled health centers through December 31, 2012

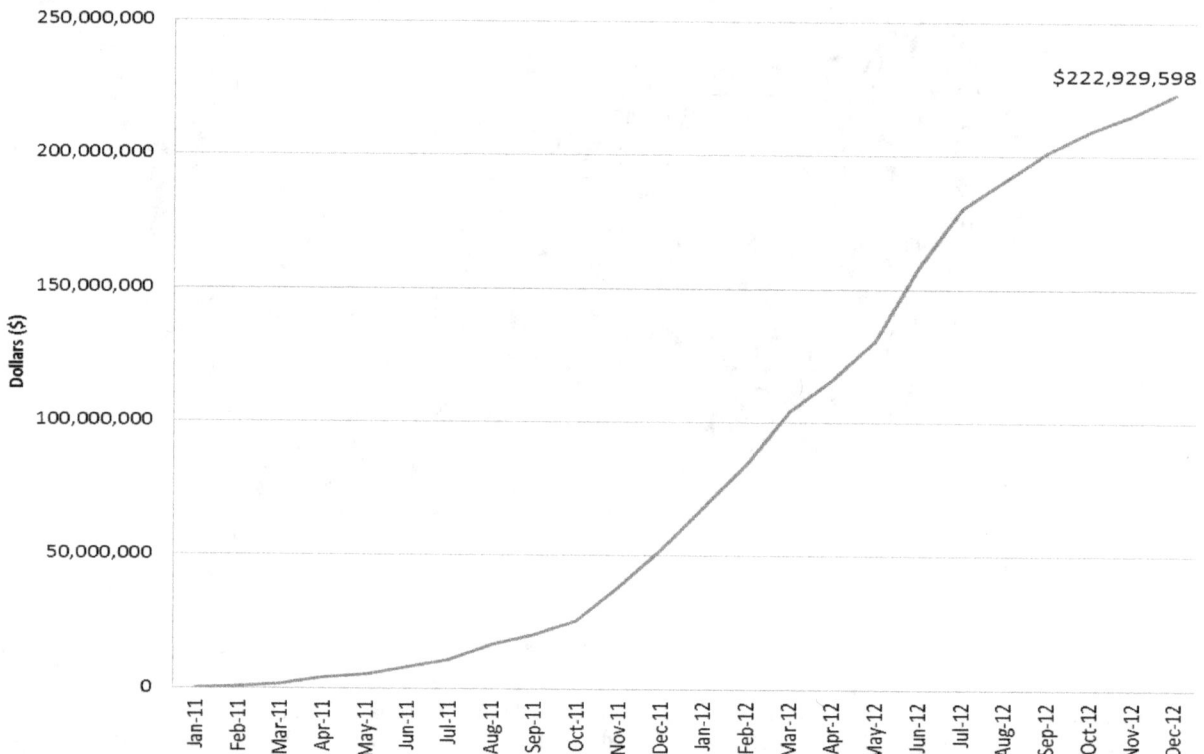

SOURCE: ONC Customer Relationship Management (CRM) Database, maintained by the Office of Provider Adoption and Support (OPAS) at ONC, and Health Care Delivery Sites list maintained by Health Resources Services Administration (HRSA). ONC CRM data as of February 18, 2013 merged with CMS EHR Incentive data through December 31, 2012.

★ 10,384 REC-assisted eligible professionals (57 percent) in health centers have received Medicaid EHR Incentive Program funds to adopt, implement or upgrade (AIU) EHR technology.

★ 798 REC-assisted eligible professionals in health centers have been paid by the Medicaid or Medicare EHR Incentive Programs for demonstrating Meaningful Use of certified EHR Technology.

RECs Enabling Care Delivery Transformation

Because health IT is an integral component to health care reform, ONC believes that the RECs are uniquely equipped to support providers' efforts use health IT to transform their delivery of care. This serves as a natural extension of their work to get providers to meaningfully use EHRs. Specifically, RECs are well positioned to continue to assist providers with the next stages of Meaningful Use (*e.g.,* Stages 2 and 3) and further develop and implement other core competencies such as privacy and security assessments, and electronic health information exchange..

RECs also continue to leverage their ability to provide technical assistance and support by working in partnership with other agencies, like CMS on priorities such as the Comprehensive Patient Care (CPC) Initiative and Accountable Care Organizations (ACOs) Programs.

Comprehensive Primary Care Initiative

ONC collaborated with the Center for Medicare & Medicaid Innovation (Innovation Center) to recruit providers for the Innovation Center's Comprehensive Primary Care Initiative, reaching out to providers that were both enrolled or not yet enrolled with the REC program. This collaboration assisted in the Innovation Center's receipt of a robust number of applicants. The Innovation Center successfully selected nearly 500 practices and over 2,300 providers into the initiative. The RECs in New Jersey, Arkansas, New York, and Cincinnati are currently working with the Innovation Center to support providers participating in the initiative in their respective markets. Additionally, the Beacon Community grantees in Cincinnati, Tulsa, and Western Colorado have also been collaborating with participants in the initiative to support practice transformation activities and enhanced use of data. The ONC and the Innovation Center continue to collaborate on opportunities to enhance technical assistance to providers in the initiative.

Accountable Care Organization (ACO) – Medicare Shared Savings Program

In April 2012, CMS announced that 27 ACOs were selected to participate in the Medicare Shared Savings Program and in July 2012, CMS announced that an additional 87 ACOs were also selected to participate in the program. In many states, these newly formed ACOs were beginning to put together plans to adopt certified EHR technology and begin measuring and reporting on electronic clinical quality measures. Several ACOs began engaging RECs for assistance related to EHR adoption, Meaningful Use, and other practice transformation and related technical assistance. With the encouragement of the ONC, RECs also engaged with ACOs to offer their services. In several cases, providers that were participating in the ACOs were previously assisted by the RECs.

With CMS' selection of an additional 106 ACOs participating in the Medicare Shared Savings Program in January 2013, ONC will be tracking continued collaboration of ACOs and RECs for health IT related technical assistance and practice transformation needs.

STATE HIE PROGRAM

Through the State Health Information Exchange (HIE) Program, ONC awarded cooperative agreements supporting health information exchange in 56 states and territories. This program has prepared states and State Designated Entities to help health care providers within their jurisdiction achieve HIE goals, objectives, and measures; that is, to ensure health information follows patients "wherever they go", regardless of organizational, vendor, or geographic boundaries.[32] As part of this overarching aim, the program has also focused on making sure that providers working to achieve Meaningful Use of health IT through Medicare and Medicaid EHR Incentive Programs have the exchange tools needed to accomplish the incentive programs' requirements. By promoting innovative approaches to the secure exchange of health information within and across states, the State HIE Program has helped grantees enable exchange services[v] in nearly every state.

Availability of Exchange Services

Directed exchange, the secure sharing of electronic health information between two known and trusted parties over networks like the internet, is a common approach that states have taken to promote exchange. Directed exchange is often less expensive to implement and operate than more complex types of exchange, and allows health care providers (and consumers) to retain control over who receives health and other personally identifiable information. Examples of cases when directed exchange is useful include when a care transition is anticipated (*e.g.,* discharge from an acute-care hospital to a long-term care setting) or when the intended recipient of information is known (*e.g.,* e-prescribing, delivery of lab results to ordering providers, a referring primary care provider sending clinical information to a specialist).

Many states have also taken measures to enable query-based exchange - that is, the ability to electronically query for and securely retrieve patient information when providers do not know the identity of other organizations and providers requiring access to patient information. Query-based exchange relies on sophisticated technology, robust policy infrastructure, and legal agreements that can sometimes be challenging to implement and maintain. Examples of cases when query-based exchange is useful include during unanticipated scenarios such as emergency department visits or when a patient goes to a healthcare provider without any accompanying medical information (*e.g.,* visits specialist without a referral).

---

[v] Most of these services are used for HIPAA-covered activities related to treatment, payment and/or operations. More specifically, health care providers often use the services to share care summaries during care transitions, send referrals, order and receive lab tests/results, look up patients' medication lists, previous diagnostic tests.

Figure 18. Directed exchange availability across the U.S. (Q4-2012)

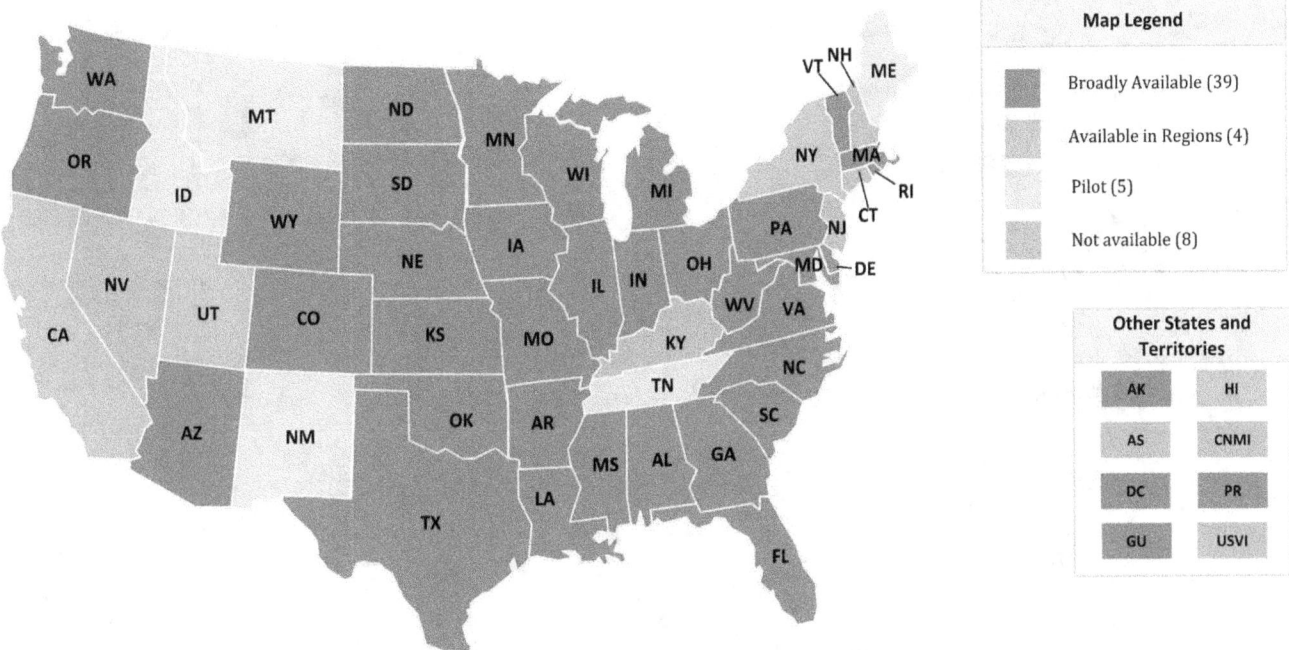

SOURCE: ONC State HIE Program Data, 2012. Estimates are aggregate self-reported information from State HIE Program grantees.

★ As of December 2012, 39 states and territories have operational directed exchange mechanisms broadly available for providers to subscribe to statewide, and nine more states have these mechanisms available in regions or as part of pilots.[vi]

[vi] *Broadly available*: Regional- and state-level entities that facilitate exchange across unaffiliated organizations exist and can be subscribed to for directed exchange. These broadly available options and services do not account for exchange enabled by enterprise (private) HIE entities serving integrated delivery networks (IDNs) or hospital systems.

* *Available in regions*: Directed exchange is available within regions of the state but not currently statewide. These options and services available in regions do not account for exchange enabled by enterprise (private) HIE entities serving IDNs or hospital systems.

* *Pilot*: Directed exchange is available to a limited number of providers participating in a pilot or test.

* *Not currently available*: Directed exchange is not yet broadly available to all providers in a state through State HIE grantee-funded or supported/enabled mechanisms. These mechanisms do not account for exchange enabled by enterprise (private) HIE entities serving IDNs or hospital systems.

Figure 19. Query exchange availability across the U.S. (Q4-2012)

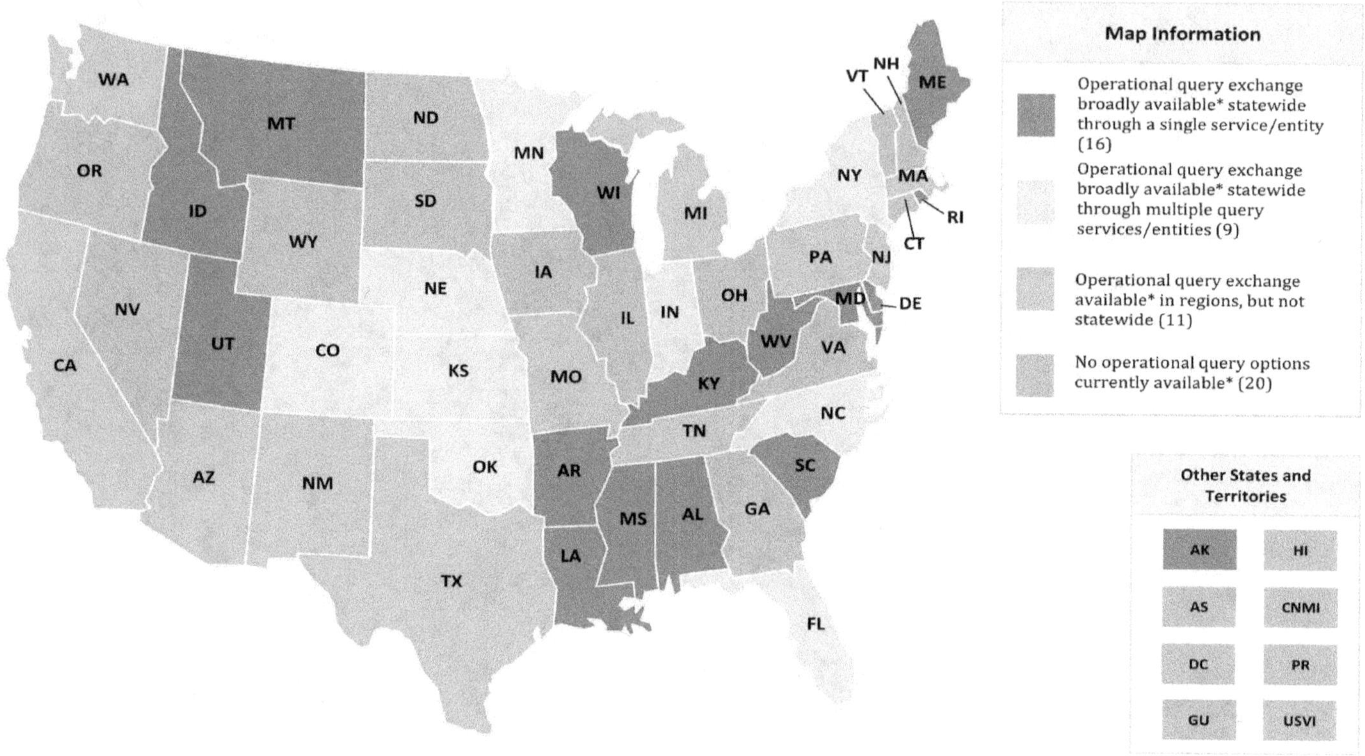

SOURCE: ONC State HIE Program Data, 2012. Estimates are aggregate self-reported information from State HIE Program grantees.

- ★ Overall, 25 states and territories have query-based exchange available to providers statewide.[vii]

  - o Specifically, in sixteen states and territories, providers can subscribe to an operational query exchange that is broadly available statewide through a single service or entity.

  - o Additionally, nine states have operational query exchange broadly available statewide through multiple query services or entities.

- ★ Eleven states have operational query exchange available in regions but not yet statewide.

[vii] *Broadly available:* Regional- and state-level entities that facilitate exchange across unaffiliated organizations exist and can be subscribed to for query-based exchange. These broadly available options and services do not account for exchange enabled by enterprise (private) HIE entities serving integrated delivery networks (IDNs) or hospital systems.

* *Available in regions*: Query-based exchange is available within regions of the state but not currently statewide. These options and services available in regions do not account for exchange enabled by enterprise (private) HIE entities serving IDNs or hospital systems.

* *Not currently available*: Query-based exchange is not yet broadly available to all providers in a state through State HIE grantee-funded or supported/enabled mechanisms. These mechanisms do not account for exchange enabled by enterprise (private) HIE entities serving IDNs or hospital systems.

Select State HIE Program Initiatives

Governance

ONC has also undertaken other initiatives to address some barriers related to cost and interoperability. ONC launched the Exemplar Health Information Exchange Governance Entities Program. This program will allow ONC to work with existing governance entities to further develop and adopt policies, interoperability requirements, and business practice criteria that align with national priorities. By advancing and further developing existing health information exchange governance models (i.e., DirectTrust.org, the EHR | HIE Interoperability Workgroup), this program promises to increase the level of secure electronic health information exchange in the nation, reduce the cost and complexity of implementation and assure the privacy and security of the electronic exchange of health information.

Consumer Mediated Exchange

In March 2012, ONC launched the Consumer Innovation Challenge (CIC), inviting interested State HIE grantees to implement innovative approaches for sharing electronic health information with consumers and enabling consumer-mediated exchange.

Georgia, Indiana, Montana, and Nebraska accepted the challenge and recently completed CIC projects. The resulting report provides a checklist of best practices for planning consumer engagement initiatives and includes information about the implementation approach, dissemination strategy, and future plans for each of the state projects.[viii]

Patient-mediated exchange is a win-win for all stakeholders. In Nebraska, the ability for consumers to download information via "Blue Button" will help providers attain Meaningful Use Stage 2 requirements in 2014. Georgia's Chatham "Connect with Direct" project is making laboratory results available to providers through the health information organization (HIO) also available to consumers, which decreases the need for providers to manage their own patient portals. In addition, equal access to information provides the opportunity for a partnership between consumer and provider, laying the groundwork for a more engaged patient.

Use partnerships and existing resources. Both Montana and Nebraska partnered with organizations have established products and services to create a new platform for patients to access their information. Montana's partners were able to incentivize consumers to sign up for the service, while Indiana was able to take advantage of a number of frameworks to execute their marketing and rollout strategy.

Successful products serve a need within the population. MyVaxIndiana has been successful in meeting a widespread recognized need for electronic access to immunization history: within four months of its launch, 14,909 total records had been accessed with usage growing each month.

Consumer demand can drive adoption. In Indiana, the MyVaxIndiana application served as a tool to encourage physicians to participate in the immunization registry system. When consumers learned they could access their immunization information any time on the internet, they asked their physicians to participate—proving that consumers have the power to drive adoption when presented with an application offering value to them. Not only has consumer enthusiasm for

---

[viii] RTI International. Consumer Innovation Challenge: Final Report. February 2013. Accessed: http://www.healthit.gov/sites/default/files/cic-paper-final.pdf

electronic access to information grown out of MyVaxIndiana's success, it has also increased interest and momentum for building new applications supported by the HIE infrastructure. The Indiana CIC project team is discussing ways the MyVaxIndiana technical framework could be used and expanded across the state.

Interoperability Modules

To support understanding and provider attainment of Stage 2 Meaningful Use requirements from the EHR Incentive Programs, the State HIE Program has developed online training tools to support grantees, eligible providers, eligible and critical access hospitals, hospitals and other stakeholders. The tools may also be useful to providers not eligible for the Medicare or Medicaid EHR Incentive Programs. The first three of the comprehensive training modules listed below have been posted on HealthIT.gov. The last two are in the process of being posted.

1. Introduction: Basics of Interoperability

2. Transitions of care between care providers and care venues

3. Lab interoperability between hospitals and ambulatory providers

4. View, download, and transmit information between patients and providers

5. Transmission of information to public health agencies

The five training modules, collectively, provide a map of Stage 2 EHR Incentive Programs' Meaningful Use attainment that help address "who, what, when and where" of achieving interoperability. ONC developed relatable use cases designed around practical workflows and provide management tools so it is easier to understand who is accountable for each element.

WORKFORCE DEVELOPMENT PROGRAM

The scarcity of a trained health IT workforce is a potential barrier to adoption of health IT. To address this problem, the Workforce Development Program seeks to train a workforce of skilled health IT professionals to help providers implement EHRs and achieve Meaningful Use. The program consists of four initiatives: Community College Consortia, Curriculum Development Centers, Competency Exam Program, and University-Based Training Program. The HITECH Workforce Development Programs have built a solid foundation of complete curricula, adaptable curricula materials, and training capacity within a network of over 90 of the nation's community colleges and universities. The programs have helped strengthen the nationwide infrastructure for providing technical assistance to the health care community as more healthcare providers move to adopt and meaningfully use EHRs.[33]

Figure 20. Number of students who successfully completed the Community College Consortia Program: February 2013

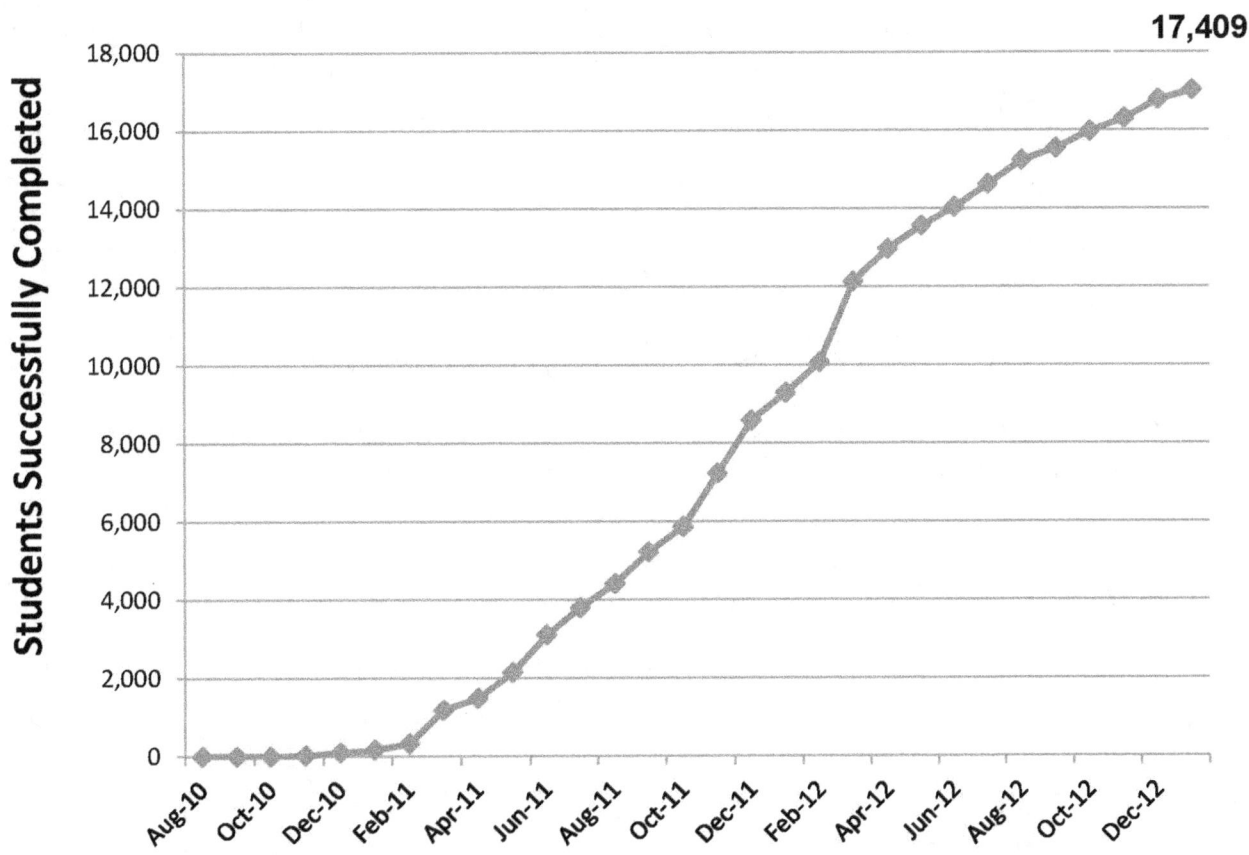

SOURCE: ONC analysis of Community College Consortia Program Data, February 2013

★ 81 colleges in five regions have collectively trained over 17,000 professionals since the launch of the Community College Consortia Program.

Figure 21. Total number of students who successfully completed the Community College Consortia Program by state as of February 2013

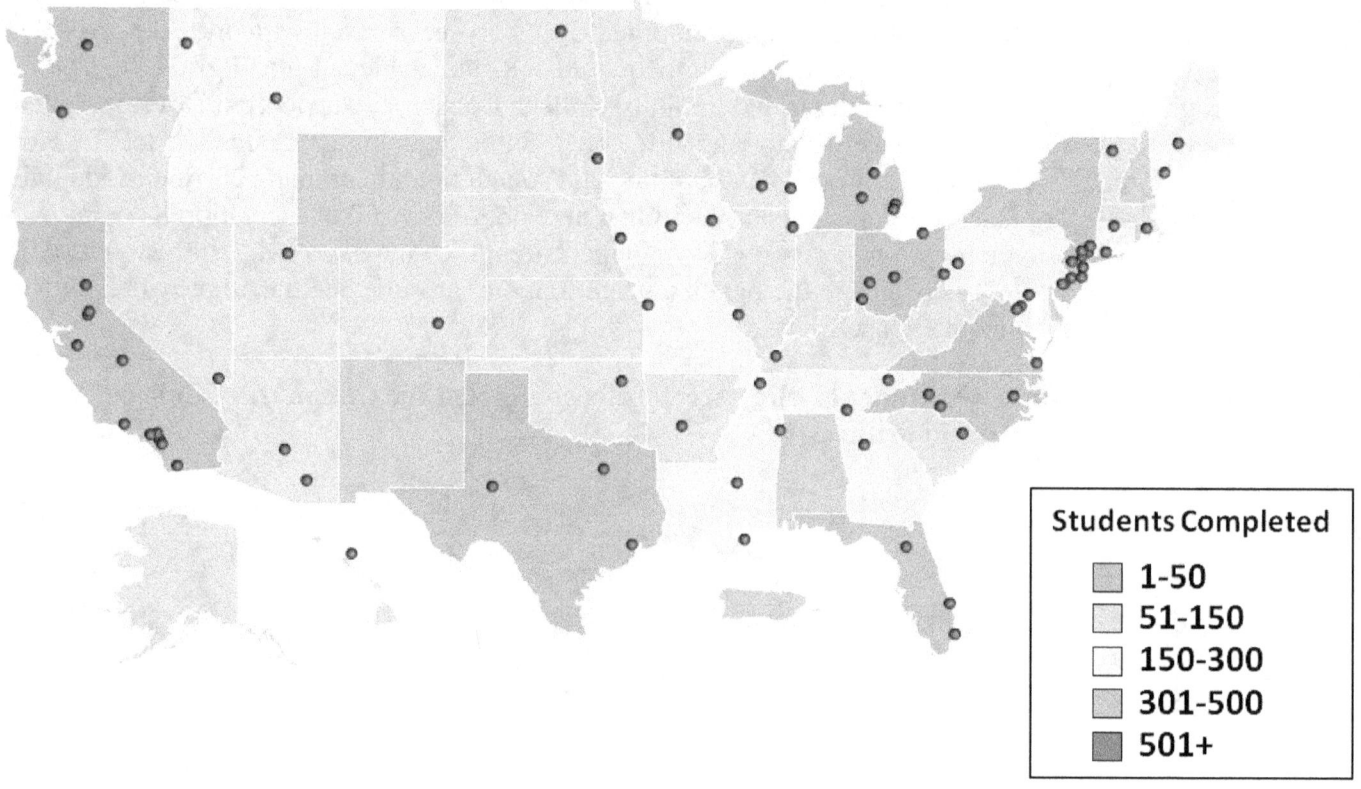

NOTES: Each point on the map represents a participating community college.
SOURCE: ONC analysis of Community College Consortia Program Data, February 2013

★ The 17,409 health IT professionals that completed Community College Consortia Program training come from every U.S. state and territory.

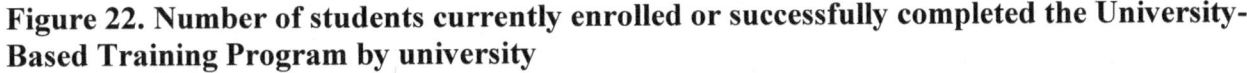

Figure 22. Number of students currently enrolled or successfully completed the University-Based Training Program by university

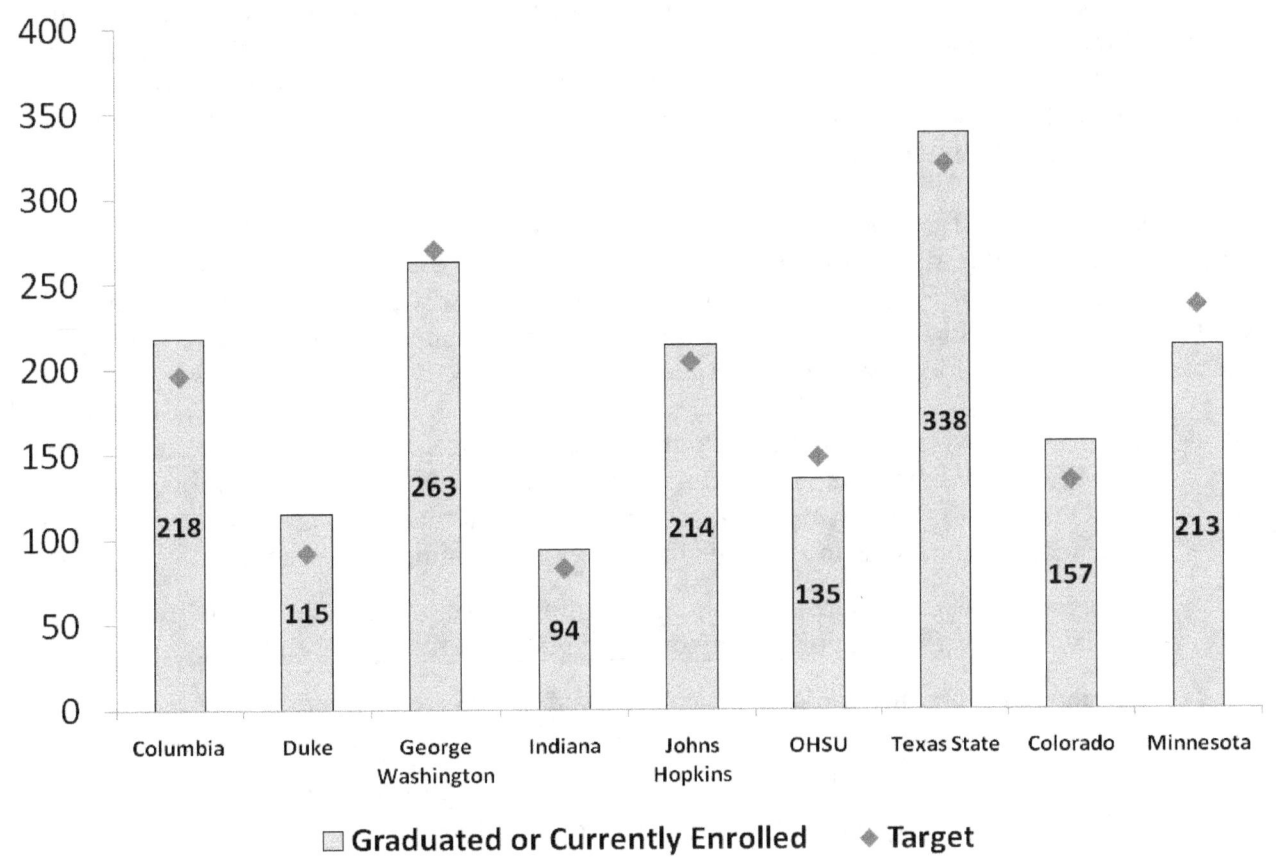

Graduated or Currently Enrolled   ◆ Target

SOURCE: ONC analysis University-Based Training Program Data, February 2013

★ The University-Based Training Program exceeded its enrollment goal of 1,685 students (1,747 students enrolled as of February 2013).

Sustainability of the Health IT Workforce Development Program

The community-college and university-based training programs initially established through ONC funding are in a position to expand and continue to meet the evolving needs of the health care environment. Beyond training students, over 10,000 individuals in more than 100 countries have downloaded materials developed by the Curriculum Development Centers. Further, more than 3,700 health IT professionals have taken exams across six workforce roles for which competency exams were developed.

The passage of the Affordable Care Act and the increasing importance of team-based care, and care coordination have started to alter the health care landscape. Educational institutions are already in the process of developing and adapting to these needs. Funding provided through the HITECH Act established a foundation of training resources that will endure and be built upon beyond the funding period. Examples include:

- The five funded Curriculum Development Centers (Oregon Health & Science University; University of Alabama at Birmingham; Johns Hopkins University; Columbia University; and Duke University) created robust training material that is now publicly available to educational institutions to start, enhance, or expand training programs.

- Bellevue College developed customized training for rural providers that is freely available (https://www.nterlearning.org/web/guest/course-details?cid=502).

- Cuyahoga Community College is using the funding to create interactive online modules for training workers to support the adoption and delivery of patient-centric care.

- Funded colleges having implemented health IT training were able to leverage other funding streams to continue to expand the training. Johnson Community College in Kansas, St. Louis Community College, St. Louis, Bellevue College, Tidewater Community College and Cuyahoga Community College were recipients of Department of Labor funding for Trade Adjustment Assistance Community College and Career Training (TAACCCT) Grants.[34]

- The competency exam will continue to be administered through the American Health Information Management Association (AHIMA) allowing health IT professionals to acquire a recognized credential that validates their knowledge, skills and abilities.

- University-Based Training grantees' new and expanded certificate and degree offerings developed through the program will continue to operate and evolve using enrollee tuition as a primary source of funding.

- Ninety percent of the funded community colleges will continue to provide industry-relevant health IT training programs. Several of the community colleges are creating career pathways between secondary and post secondary education and developing articulation agreements between colleges and universities.

BEACON COMMUNITY PROGRAM

The Beacon Community Cooperative Agreement Program demonstrates how health IT investments and Meaningful Use of EHRs advance the vision of patient-centered care, while improving quality and lowering costs of care. ONC awarded $250 million over three years to 17 selected communities throughout the United States that have demonstrated progress in the development of secure, private, and accurate systems of EHR use and health information exchange. As of the end of 2012, over 8,700 providers are participating in Beacon Communities, affecting over 8 million lives. Each of the 17 communities—with its unique population and regional context—is actively pursuing the following areas of focus:

- Building and strengthening the health IT infrastructure and exchange capabilities within communities, positioning each community to pursue a new level of sustainable health care quality and efficiency over the coming years;

- Translating investments in health IT to measureable improvements in cost, quality and population health, and;

- Developing innovative approaches to performance measurement, technology and care delivery to accelerate evidence generation for new approaches.

Figure 23. Location of Beacon Communities

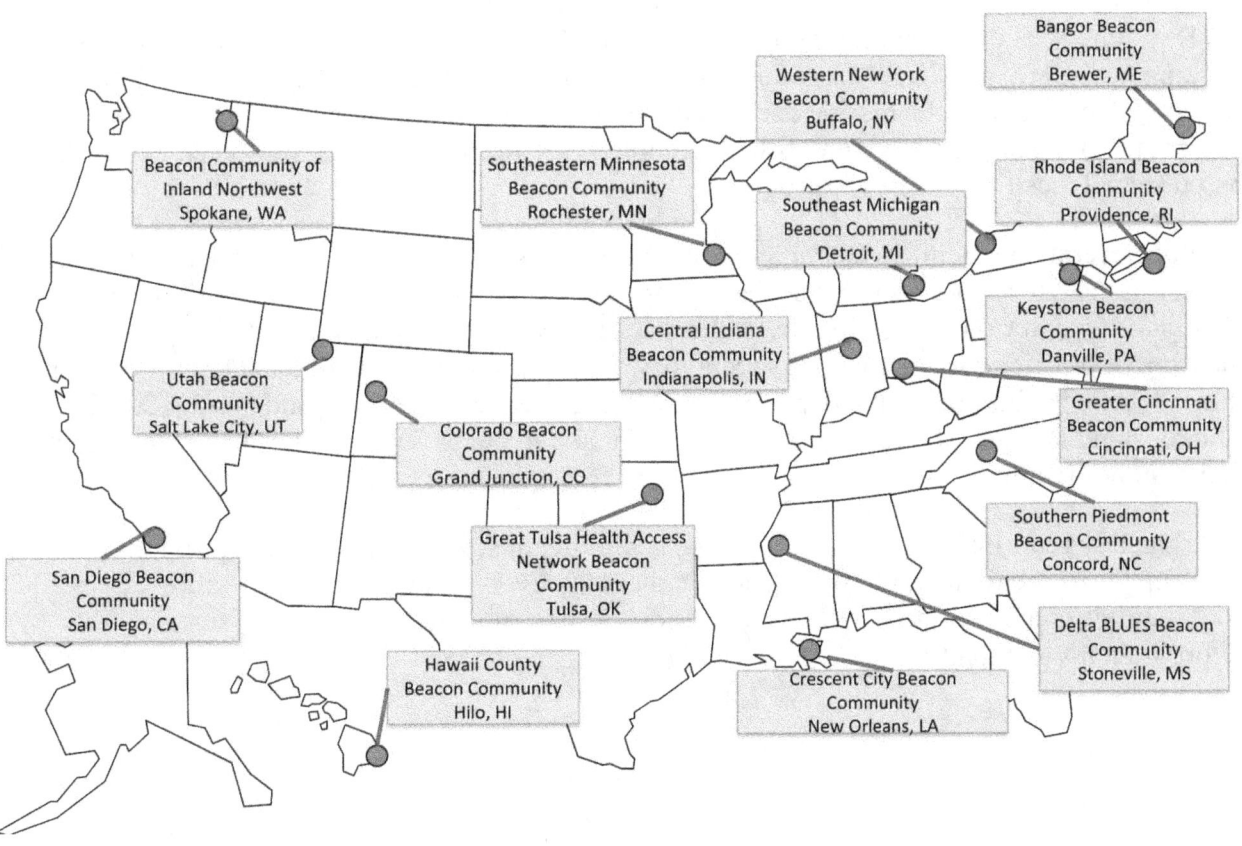

Beacon communities have taken major steps to build and strengthen their health IT infrastructure to enable the fluid transmission of data across their communities. During the three-year grant period, seven communities established capabilities to exchange health information (MN, MI, RI, OK, CA, MS, LA). Additionally, five communities are using technology to build partnerships with public health agencies (CA, MN, NC, NY, UT) and four communities have built partnerships with home health and skilled nursing facilities to improve transitions of care (ME, NY, RI, PA). Thirteen communities are testing innovative tools and strategies to deliver patient-centered care including: mobile health (CA, LA, MI, OH, UT); tele-monitoring (CA, IN, ME, MN, NY); personalized clinical decision support (CO, OK); and EHRs (NY, PA).

Several communities show improving care for chronic diseases including cardiovascular disease, diabetes and asthma. For example, between Q4-2010 and Q4-2012, the Bangor Beacon Community improved LDL-C Control for patients with cardiovascular disease from 57 percent to 65 percent. And, between Q2-2011 and Q4-2012, the Crescent City Beacon Community improved diabetes HbA1c control rates from 50 percent to 59 percent within their initial group of three clinics; and from 45 percent to 52 percent within their second wave subsequent cohort of ten clinics.

Communities are also focused on reducing costly unnecessary hospital utilizations, including emergency department visits, hospital admissions and readmissions. The Bangor Beacon Community decreased the rate of hospital admissions from 26 percent to 16 percent and the emergency department visit rate from 26 percent to 17 percent; among its "high risk/high cost" patient cohort that completed 12 months of care management. Between Q1-2011 and Q2-2012, the Keystone Beacon Community improved 30-day readmission rate among KBC-managed patients with CHF and COPD from 25 percent to 16 percent. And, in Q4-2012, San Diego Beacon Community Collaborative decreased the 30-day inpatient readmission rate from 18 percent to 13 percent among patients with complex care needs through a four-week evidence-based Care Transitions Initiative program.

Finally, several communities are targeting improvements in population health measures, like screening rates for depression. Since the beginning of the Beacon intervention period, the Colorado Beacon Consortium improved depression screening for patients with diabetes within their initial practice cohort from 55 percent to 85 percent of patients with diabetes within their initial practice cohort receiving depression screening. Between Q2-2011 and Q4-2012, the Rhode Island Beacon Community improved from 50 percent to 85 percent of patients receiving depression screening.

Over the last year, Beacon Communities made significant strides to use their health IT investments as the foundation for payment and care delivery innovation. Many more communities continue to make these connections as part of a larger health care sustainability effort in their community.

HEALTH IT CERTIFICATION PROGRAM

In FY 2010, ONC developed and implemented a temporary certification program, authorized six ONC-Authorized Testing and Certification Bodies (ONC-ATCBs), and established the Certified Health IT Products List (CHPL) to assure providers eligible for EHR incentives that the products they purchase would be able to support their achievement of Meaningful Use under Medicare and Medicaid EHR Incentive Programs. ONC collaborated with the National Institute of Standards and Technology (NIST) to develop test procedures to assess EHRs ability to perform capabilities in a manner that is standards compliant.

The Temporary Certification Program became operational in Q1-FY2011 and sunset roughly a year later as ONC launched the ONC HIT Certification Program (formally referred to as the Permanent Certification Program). As of February 2013, 937 vendors sought certification of 3,052 EHR technology products. Based upon earlier analyses of the CHPL list and CMS EHR Incentive Program data, more than three quarters (77 percent) of vendors provided certified electronic health record technology (CEHRT) products for use by eligible professionals, 15 percent of vendors provided CEHRT products for use by eligible hospitals, and the remaining vendors provided CEHRT products for use by both eligible professionals and hospitals.[35]

ONC in collaboration with American National Standards Institute (ANSI) and National Voluntary Laboratory Accreditation Program (NVLAP) has authorized scope expansion for Authorized Testing Laboratories (ATLs) and ONC-Authorized Certification Bodies (ONC-ACBs) for the 2014 Edition EHR certification criteria in Q1-FY2013. ONC continues to monitor stakeholder experience with the 2014 Edition Test Method, in collaboration with the NIST.

ONC has worked closely with CMS in the development of clinical quality measures that enable providers to better understand their performance relative to quality standards. In addition, ONC has developed a rigorous testing platform as a component of our 2014 EHR technology certification program that requires that every EHR capture the data necessary to compute clinical quality measures, calculate the measures accurately, and report the results of that calculation in a standard way to CMS.

PRIVACY & SECURITY

The position of ONC's Chief Privacy Officer was created to advise the National Coordinator on privacy, security, and data stewardship of electronic health information and to coordinate with the HHS Office for Civil Rights (OCR), other Federal agencies, state and regional efforts, and with foreign countries with regard to the privacy, security, and data stewardship of electronic individually identifiable health information (eIIHI). ONC's Chief Privacy Officer, in coordination with OCR has developed a flexible, iterative process for assessing, prioritizing, and implementing privacy and security-related initiatives. This includes providing guidance regarding how the HIPAA Privacy and Security Rules can facilitate the implementation of EHRs and addressing concerns regarding privacy and security issues. ONC addresses these issues through a multi-pronged approach that includes targeted technical assistance materials, provider education, assistance, and outreach, and pilot projects that test new technological solutions to enhance patient choice and control over the sharing of eIIHI while removing implementation barriers, and targeted program guidance.

In 2012, ONC's Office of the Chief Privacy Officer (OCPO) efforts were focused on influencing major regulatory activities impacting the privacy and security of eIIHI, such as the Affordable Care Act regulations and EHR Incentive Programs Stage 2 regulations, as well as addressing a primary threat to eIIHI – the loss or theft of computing devices, and in particular portable devices. Additionally, OCPO implemented key Health IT Policy Committee and Health IT Standards Committee recommendations, developed and provided technical assistance information, and continued to work across federal agencies, and participate in internationally focused efforts, in order to address and help safeguard the privacy and security of health information.

Regulatory activity

- OCPO, in coordination with OCR, reviewed and contributed to the Affordable Care Act regulations, ensuring that privacy, security, and data stewardship policies were appropriately incorporated into the final rules governing the new modes for exchanging and analyzing health information under the Affordable Care Act. This effort addressed regulations governing: accountable care organizations; qualified entities that provide performance measurement services, and the health insurance marketplace.

- OCPO reviewed and contributed to regulations for Stage 2 Meaningful Use for the EHR Incentive Programs by reviewing the regulations to see that they would adequately protect health information by requiring providers and hospitals, as a condition of receiving incentive payments, to attest that they have conducted a security risk assessment, specifically addressing encryption of data at rest, implemented security updates, and corrected security deficiencies that were identified.

Cross Agency/International activity

- OCPO provided health sector input and perspective to The National Science & Technology Council (NSTC)'s Subcommittee on Privacy and Internet Policy for the development of the White House Internet Privacy Policy, *Consumer Data Privacy in a Networked World.*

- OCPO, in coordination with the State Department and the HHS Office of Global Affairs, provided input on the U.S. government's response to the European Commission's proposed Data Protection Regulation.

- OCPO is involved in the national effort to use the Veterans Affairs Department's Blue Button technology to offer more than 80 million citizens the ability to download their electronic health care records. OCPO is working closely with federal policymakers to assure that the data are protected and secure while supporting the right that individuals have under the HIPAA Privacy Rule to review and obtain a copy of their health information electronic form.

- OCPO supported the Data Segmentation for Privacy Initiative (DS4P), which, through collaboration among federal and industry partners identify innovative ways of protecting the privacy of health information. The DS4P initiative has explored a number of standards that prevent health information from being inappropriately shared between different entities, and has drafted an implementation guide to help providers withhold certain sensitive health information when sharing it would not be appropriate. The DS4P initiative launched three pilot programs to test the implementation guide and provide feedback and recommendations for possible action by the Health IT Policy and Standards Committees.

Initiatives related to portable devices and health information

- OCPO, in conjunction with OCR hosted a successful (1,000+ participants) public roundtable and comment period on securing and protecting health information while using mobile devices across various health care delivery settings. The result of the roundtable and comment period public input was the development and release of an educational initiative and resource center for those in the clinical sector on how to protect and secure health information when using a mobile device.

- OCPO developed testing protocols to analyze popular mobile devices (smart phones, tablets, and laptop computers) to determine security measures needed to keep health information secured on mobile devices. This resulted in the development of:

  o An assessment of mobile devices currently on the market to determine if they have security features built in that would assist in compliance with NIST and HITECH standards that an individual could manually enable "out of the box" to protect health information accessed or stored on the device.

  o Suggested ways to configure the devices to improve "out of the box" security. These device-specific guidelines will soon be publicly available on HealthIT.gov.

- In FY 2012, OCPO engaged in data gathering activities to further identify the issues surrounding mobile health by conducting a series of focus groups to identify and explore consumer attitudes, concerns and preferences on the privacy and security of health-related information communicated via mobile devices in. In FY 2013, ONC plans to release a report on this information and share results.

Other key efforts

- OCPO reviewed the Health IT Policy Committee recommendations on privacy and security safeguards and health information exchange, particularly those relevant to offering individuals' the choice of whether to participate in certain types of electronic health information exchange, and furthered the adoption of these recommendations through the release of the State HIE Privacy and Security Program Instruction Notice to grantees.

- OCPO initiated an eConsent pilot project to develop, pilot, and evaluate innovative ways to meaningfully inform individuals of their options with respect to the sharing of their electronic health information and to electronically capture an individual's choice.

- OCPO fielded a national survey to measure consumer privacy and security concerns. This survey reports on consumer perceptions to examine their perspectives on safeguarding health information and help gauge progress with regards to ONC's goal "to inspire confidence and trust in health IT." Subsequent rounds of the survey will enable examining changes in consumer perceptions over time.

- OCPO developed privacy and security oriented technical assistance materials for ONC grantees and other stakeholders. Such materials included the *Cybersecure Your Medical Practice* video game to help providers train their employees on general security practices to safeguard ePHI and resources, addressing the security of ePHI when using mobile devices.

- OCPO provided ongoing management of the Strategic Health IT Advanced Research Project for Security (SHARP-S) grant, which encompasses a series of research projects focused on the following areas: Audit Management, Integrity Management, Media Management, Access Management, and Security Program Management. The privacy and security solutions developed under the SHARP-S grant are intended to move the marketplace forward and inform policy development.

- OCPO reviewed and had significant input into development of the Workforce Development Program's nationally available curricular materials related to privacy and security.

Upcoming activities

In FY 2014, OCPO anticipates that new privacy and security policy issues will arise due to the increasing adoption of EHRs by health care providers and the participation of more diverse entities in health information exchange. Additionally, the rapid change in technologies impacting health information systems creates ongoing privacy and security issues, as does the growing globalization of health care and research. And finally, privacy and security will remain critical issues to address in the development and implementation of health insurance marketplaces and accountable care organizations.

ONC will address upcoming privacy and security priorities, including those referenced above, through the following activities:

- Focus on identifying and addressing cybersecurity threats;

- Providing and disseminating technical assistance in areas (including but not limited to) Security Program Management, Risk Management, Access Management, Integrity Management, Audit Management, Incident Management, Continuity Management, Chains of Trust Controls, Workforce Management, and Media Management;

- Work with NIST and other partners to assure that correct clinical information is associated with the correct patients and / or providers by supporting innovative frameworks that can provide a foundation for identity management;

- Continuing to incorporate policy components that further privacy and security in future stages of Meaningful Use; and,

- Continuing work on patient and provider identity management

ONC's Office of Science and Technology (OST) works to enable development and use of interoperability standards that enable health data to be accurately collected, securely exchanged, and effectively used by health IT products and services on which health professionals and consumers rely. The progression of Meaningful Use requirements from data collection to electronic health information exchange and demonstrating improved processes, coordination and outcomes of care depends on the specification of standards, services, and policies that support interoperability and exchange of electronic health information. ONC supports the development of health IT standards through the standards and interoperability framework, existing standards development organizations and the Federal Health Architecture. OST standards and interoperability efforts engage the private sector as well as federal, state, local, and tribal government entities in efforts to incrementally but steadily advance the prevalence of seamless, secure use and exchange of health data amongst and between all stakeholders.

ONC's OST is responsible for a portfolio of activities critical to advancing an environment of the seamless exchange of health information in a private and secure manner. These activities result in ONC providing for a core set of needed publicly accessible specifications, tools, and services that support interoperability, exchange, and use of standardized electronic health information. These activities include:

- Supporting the life-cycle of standards and implementation specifications for health IT, including testing and implementation of existing and new standards that support information exchange and use;

- Identifying, where possible, existing standards, service descriptions, and implementation specifications for health IT to meet priority health policy goals;

- Supporting, where needed, the development of new standards, service descriptions, and implementation specifications for health IT to meet priority health policy goals;

- Coordinating federal participation in health information exchange (e.g., through the Federal Health Architecture);

- Supporting a presidential priority initiative to enable health information exchange between the Department of Defense and Department of Veterans Affairs, which will benefit care coordination, quality, and outcomes for military personnel, dependents, and veterans;

- Leveraging an innovative challenges and prizes mechanism[ix] to create and disperse tools among the developer community in order to promote and advance health IT interoperability and health information exchange objectives.

- Developing and promoting standards to facilitate the emergence of systems and services whereby shareable CDS interventions through the Health eDecisions initiative.

[ix] One of the first new prize and challenge programs to become operational under the government-wide authority established by the America COMPETES Reauthorization Act of 2010 (P.L. 111-358).

ONC's high-level approach to meeting these responsibilities and fostering interoperable health IT products and systems includes:

- **Supporting flexible, incremental, and modular standards:** ONC has not attempted to develop a centralized or "top down" approach to interoperability. Instead, through the Standards & Interoperability (S&I) Framework, ONC supports the development of flexible, modular standards and harmonizes a portfolio of standards, services, and policies that provide flexible ways for different systems in different settings to interact and exchange information with one another.

- **Selecting standards that work for the future:** ONC's work advancing interoperability continually and deliberately considers the need for the health IT infrastructure to be adaptable, so that it can meet today's needs but still accommodate new policy, payment models and technology in the future. For example, ONC has made empowering consumers and patients a central part of our strategy to increase information exchange. Using existing standards from the ONC standards portfolio, ONC was able to support the broader community's develop new functionality that leveraged standards for vocabularies, documents, and transport that empowers patients to view, download and transmit their medical records information to a personal health record.

- **Make incremental changes with community feedback:** ONC takes an incremental, iterative approach that engages the community to help identify problems and quickly develop new solutions. ONC uses feedback from real-world pilots to help refine and improve the standards available for health information interoperability and exchange.

- **Supporting implementation and pre-certification testing:** Health IT interoperability standards, specifications, and services are successful when vendors, providers and others are able to effectively, efficiently implement and use these resources. Supporting implementation and pre-certification testing efforts is critical both to learning that helps to accelerate incremental improvement of interoperability resources and to helping the health IT vendor and user communities succeed in information exchange and use.

The cornerstone of this approach comprises the ONC-led Standards and Interoperability (S&I) Framework and Implementation and Standards Implementation & Testing (I&T) Platform efforts, which focus on driving standards development and supporting interoperability and exchange of electronic health information exchange.

The S&I Framework is an example of "government as a platform for innovation" through which ONC engages the technical expertise of individuals in the health IT vendor and user communities to identify and develop solutions to practical challenges faced in efforts to use nationally recognized standards to achieve interoperability. The Framework supports the community by providing a forum and collaboration tools to help these individuals develop and test solutions to these challenges that can be successfully used throughout the nation. Solutions developed often include new or revised detailed technical standards or standards-implementation reference information. Since its inception in early 2011, more than 700 people have participated in over 1,500 S&I Framework working sessions, and over 1,500 more have registered to observe and participate less intensively through the S&I Framework's wiki. Prior to the S&I Framework, development of new or significantly revised standards typically took 18-36 months. Within the S&I Framework, the process can be routinely completed in only 9-18 months.

The Standards Implementation & Testing (I&T) Platform efforts launched after the S&I Framework, to complement the S&I Framework by advancing two related goals: supporting implementers in their efforts to use nationally recognized standards to achieve interoperability and exchange of electronic health information; and enabling ONC to rapidly gather information on challenges encountered, and strategies deployed to address these challenges, by implementers using standards such as the HL-7 Consolidated Clinical Document Architecture (C-CDA) in the field. The I&T Platform serves as a resource for identifying implementers' knowledge needs and for disseminating knowledge to support the effective implementation and, as necessary, ongoing development of health information standards to support seamless, secure exchange.

FEDERAL HEALTH ARCHITECTURE

The Federal Health Architecture (FHA) has implemented a new Strategic Plan for 2013-2015 to better support the needs of its federal partners and health information exchange efforts across the federal space. The document represents a collection of ideas from FHA partner working sessions and individual FHA partner interviews. The vision for FHA is "a federal health information technology environment that is interoperable with the private sector and supports the President's health information technology plan enabling better care, increased efficiency, and improved population health." In order to reach that vision, FHA has adopted the following three strategic goals with key supporting objectives:

- **Goal 1**: Improve exchange of health data among the federal government, private sector healthcare providers and other appropriate stakeholders, by establishing a unified federal voice on health data exchange interoperability.

   o Objective 1.1: Establish the FHA partnership as the "convener of stature," a comprehensive forum for all government agencies involved in healthcare data exchange.

   o Objective 1.2: Institutionalize governance decision-making processes.

   o Objective 1.3: Conduct outreach to collect best practices and coordinate implementation.

- **Goal 2**: Encourage adoption of interoperability specifications, resulting in active data exchange in the Federal health community.

   o Objective 2.1: Support the Standards and Interoperability (S&I) Framework Initiatives by providing federal use cases (which inform S&I Framework activities' evolution of standards) and encouraging implementation of standards at FHA partner agencies.

   o Objective 2.2: Use Federal Health Architecture to enable partners to move from legacy to new solutions in an efficient, coordinated manner.

- **Goal 3**: Align federal policies in health data exchange to use the federal government's combined influence as a payer, provider, and public health guardian to improve the healthcare system.

o Objective 3.1: Serve as a forum for cataloging and aligning federal policies and practices as they apply to interoperability.

A significant achievement of FHA over the past year was the open-source release, in February 2013, of version 4.0 of the CONNECT software[x] that uses recognized, vendor-neutral health data standards to enable electronic health information exchange. Initially developed by federal agencies to support their health-related missions, CONNECT is now available to all organizations, and can be used to help enable HIE and share data using nationally recognized interoperability standards. This version of CONNECT, supports current federal IT standards and Meaningful Use Stage 2 core objectives related to the secure electronic exchange of information through CONNECT's support of Direct Project specifications and Nationwide Health Information Network (NwHIN) transports (*i.e.,* electronically sending and receiving patient data, registering immunization information, public health reporting and patient access to data). CONNECT 4.0 also offers users improved flexibility through its modular platform that allows users to pick and choose which components they want to use in their IT environment. FHA's ultimate goal is to fully transition maintenance of CONNECT to the open source community where it can continue to evolve to better support safe, effective, well-coordinated and accessible care.

Also within the past year, FHA sponsored an open-source, exploratory project in RESTful Health Exchange (RHEx) that demonstrated simple, secure, standards-based web technologies for health information exchange. Continuing the tradition of federal partner investment to find and share with the entire health IT community solutions to their health IT needs, RHEx leveraged the S&I Framework approach and infrastructure to complete projects designed to inform a path forward toward availability of health information exchange approaches that could use Representational State Transfer (REST) technology to complement existing health information exchange mechanisms.

eHEALTH EXCHANGE

The Nationwide Health Information Network (NwHIN) Exchange has been renamed to eHealth Exchange and its operation has transitioned to a public-private partnership, as of October 2012. The eHealth Exchange is composed of federal agencies and private-sector partners that have implemented NwHIN standards and services, and executed the Data Use and Reciprocal Support Agreement (DURSA) legal agreement, in order to securely exchange electronic health information. The Exchange Coordinating Committee that oversees eHealth Exchange has designated Healtheway, a nonprofit organization, to assume operational support of eHealth Exchange. Healtheway will support eHealth Exchange with conformance and interoperability testing, onboarding of new participants, and maintenance of the DURSA, operating policies and procedures, the service registry and digital certificates. This transition to a public-private partnership reflects ONC's strategy to be an "incubator" for innovation and its focus on supporting a sustainable ecosystem of organizations using secure and scalable ways to exchange health information.

---

[x] The CONNECT software and information supporting its use is available via the CONNECT Community Portal at http://www.connectopensource.org.

CONSUMER eHEALTH

Patient and family engagement is increasingly recognized as a key component of many efforts to transform the health care system and achieve better population health. One of the five goals of the *Federal Health IT Strategic Plan* is to "empower individuals with health IT to improve their health and the health care system."[36] This goal recognizes the important role that patients and their caregivers play in determining their health outcomes. Patients and their caregivers often coordinate care among multiple providers, decide whether and when to seek health care services, and are ultimately responsible for health-related behaviors ranging from taking medications to managing diet and exercise.

Giving patients both access to their health information electronically and electronic tools and services for using that information can better position them to participate more fully in their care; self manage their health conditions; coordinate care across multiple providers; and improve communication with their care teams—those directly involved in their care. Consumer eHealth tools and services, such as personal health records, mobile apps, and remote monitoring devices can empower and support consumers to manage their health on their own, or in coordination with their care team.

The role of ONC in advancing consumer eHealth is primarily as a catalyst and convener, providing incentives, supporting others—such as patients, providers, and technology developers—who are at the forefront of advancing consumer engagement via eHealth. ONC has developed the "Three A's" strategy to fulfill its goal. The three prongs of the strategy are to increase patients' ability to *access* their health information electronically; enable consumers to take *action* using their health information; and to shift *attitudes* so patients and providers think and act as partners in managing health and healthcare using health IT and eHealth tools.

ONC participates in numerous initiatives that contribute to meeting these objectives, including:

- Increasing consumer *access* to their electronic health information through outreach and support to organizations that have voluntarily taken the Blue Button Pledge and committed to implementing "Blue Button"—providing a way for individuals to view and download their health data electronically, and educating consumers about the benefit of accessing their health data electronically. The Pledge Program now includes more than 450 organizations. ONC is also working to equip providers with tools to assist in meeting Stage 2 Meaningful Use requirements for eligible providers and hospitals that require them to enable patients by providing a way for patients to view, download and transmit their health information to a third party. Under this provision patients will be able to export their data from EHRs in structured, machine-readable, and human readable formats and to share that data with others. ONC collaborated with more than 68 organizations through the Standards & Interoperability Framework "Automate Blue Button" to develop and publish an implementation guide for data holders and developers on Blue Button+, which meets and builds on these Meaningful Use requirements.

- Catalyzing the development of innovative consumer health IT tools and resources to help consumers take *action* with their health data, by funding application developer contests to spur market innovation in the area of consumer health applications focused on addressing a health priority or area of need that aligns with federal health priorities and is not already

---

being addressed by private sector innovation. Recent challenges include the Health Record Design contest that invited designers to rethink how the medical record is presented visually; and a Blue Button Mash-Up Challenge to create mobile applications that combine an individual's Blue Button health data with other types of data to make the information more usable and meaningful. ONC also completed a pilot at Geisinger Health System to evaluate the role of patients in improving the accuracy of the information in their medical records, which revealed that patient feedback is valuable and improves the accuracy and completeness of that information.

- Shifting *attitudes* about the role of patients and providers as partners in care by developing tools and guidance on specific ways consumers can use technology to manage their health and expand current outreach efforts to target individuals with chronic disease and the underserved. The HHS Office for Civil Rights recently launched a campaign to build public awareness of individuals' legal right to access their health information under the HIPAA Privacy Rule. Through HealthIT.gov, ONC is serving as a one-stop shop for information about health IT, eHealth tools ,and profiles about patient stories about how using these tools and getting engaged in health is impacting people's lives. In 2012, ONC ran a series of video contests encouraging the public to share their person stories and developed an animated video to make learning about health IT and the power of having online access to health data fun and accessible.

In 2013, ONC will continue to refine and realize a vision in which the individual patient or consumer is at the center of their own health and health care, supported by health IT. ONC will continue to push to increase the percentage of Americans that have secure, electronic access to their health information and the number of individuals who actually use that information to manage their health and coordinate their care. ONC will also work to provide the policy and technical building blocks needed to achieve such a vision, by tracking and responding to trends, such as the growing role of social media in health, the growing interest in patient generated health data, the analysis and application of health information from various sources.

ONC worked collaboratively with colleagues throughout the HHS to develop the Health IT Patient Safety Action and Surveillance Plan, which was released on December 21, 2012. This Health IT Safety Plan addresses the role of health IT within HHS' commitment to patient safety. The draft plan prescribes actions that all stakeholders can take within their existing authorities and resources to promote a culture of safety related to health IT.

CLINICAL DECISION SUPPORT

Clinical decision support (CDS) provides clinicians, staff, patients, or other individuals with knowledge and person-specific information, intelligently filtered or presented at appropriate times, to enhance health and health care. CDS encompasses computerized alerts and reminders to care providers and patients, clinical guidelines, condition-focused order sets, patient data reports and summaries, documentation templates, diagnostic support, and other tools that enhance decision making in clinical workflow.

CDS is critical to advancing health IT-enabled clinical quality improvement, and is a core component of the EHR Incentive Programs' requirements. ONC is committed to promoting the advancement of clinical decision support to support the triple aim. ONC has facilitated a variety of activities to catalyze progress in CDS development and deployment in support of enhanced health and care, including:

- **Advancing Clinical Decision Support (ACDS):** Completed in early 2012, ACDS was a multi-part project funded by ONC to address the major barriers to achieving widespread use of clinical decision support through four tasks. The tasks were: preparing resources on best practices for broad dissemination; produce an open online platform for sharing CDS knowledge artifacts (such as alerts, order sets, etc.) among EHR vendors and/or provider organizations; develop a "clinically important" drug-drug interaction (DDI) list, as well as a legal brief about the liability implications of using the clinically important DDI list; develop a process that engages specialty bodies in weighing performance gaps vs. CDS opportunities to select targets for meaningful use of CDS by specialists.

- **Ongoing support for and coordination of the CDS Federal Collaboratory:** a federal community of interest, formed in 2008 to focus on CDS as a key health information technology component for improving the quality, safety, efficiency and effectiveness of health care.

- **Health eDecisions (HeD):** Within the S&I Framework, the Health eDecisions initiative is working to identify, define and harmonize standards that facilitate the emergence of systems and services whereby shareable CDS interventions can be implemented to facilitate integration of a system with CDS interventions via:

  - Standards to structure medical knowledge in a shareable and executable format for use in CDS, and
  - Standards that define how a system can interact with and utilize an electronic interface that provides helpful, actionable clinical guidance

  In order to facilitate integration of a system with CDS interventions, the scope includes standards to refer to data in electronic health records and standards to map recommendations to locally implementable actions.

- **Strategic Health IT Advanced Research Projects SHARP C:** SHARP C focuses on Patient-Centered Cognitive Support to harness the power of health IT to integrate and support physician reasoning and decision-making as providers care for patients.

BARRIERS TO ADOPTION OF HEALTH INFORMATION TECHNOLOGY

KEY BARRIERS TO EHR ADOPTION FACED BY OFFICE-BASED PHYSICIANS

The top barriers to EHR adoption reported across a nationally representative survey of office-based physicians who provide direct patient care are concerned about the cost of purchasing an EHR system and have concerns regarding loss of productivity (Table 8). Those who have yet to adopt an EHR system express significantly higher level of concerns regarding the potential barriers compared to EHR adopters who report the actual barriers they have experienced. Additionally, at least 4 in 10 physicians who have yet to adopt EHRs also express concerns regarding EHR maintenance costs, selecting an EHR that meets their practices needs, adequacy of technical support and practice resistance. These results include all office-based physicians and are not limited to eligible professionals.

Key HITECH programs address many barriers experienced by EHR adopters as well as concerns raised by those who have yet to adopt EHRs, including the provision of financial incentives to support adoption and Meaningful Use of EHRs and the REC Program, which focuses on assisting providers with EHR adoption and Meaningful Use of EHRs.

Table 8. Barriers to EHR adoption by adoption status

	Adopters	Nonadopters	Difference
Cost of purchasing a system	52	73	21*
Loss of productivity	37	59	22*
Effort needed to select a system	28	38	11*
Adequacy of training	27	41	14*
Annual maintenance cost	26	46	20*
Finding an EHR that meets practice needs	26	45	20*
Adequacy of technical support	25	40	15*
Resistance of practice to change work habits	22	40	19*
Reliability of the system	15	40	25*
Ability to secure financing	14	29	15*
Reaching consensus within the practice	10	18	8*
Access to high speed Internet	9	7	(1)

* Significant difference between adopter and nonadopter (p<0.01). Numbers may not add up due to rounding.
SOURCE: NCHS Physician Workflow Survey, 2011.

ADDRESSING CHALLENGES TO EHR ADOPTION: THE ROLE OF RECS

The REC program monitors and addresses key challenges to EHR adoption and achieving Meaningful Use faced by providers that are participating in the program. The REC program has placed a great emphasis on sharing information (knowledge transfer) and lessons learned to help address barriers. Specifically the Health Information Technology Research Center (HITRC) and National Learning Consortium (NLC) identify best practices and facilitate shared learning through communities of practice. The support they provide to address barriers includes:

- Technical expertise to assist RECs in their efforts to recruit and educate providers

- Development of tools and trainings to assist providers with effective vendor selection processes, workflow redesign techniques, project management and achieving Meaningful Use. To date, the RECs have provided 69 reports, 836 tools, and 138 presentations.

- There were over 400,000 hits in 2012 alone to the HITRC Portal page that provides technical assistance.

- The REC program organizes and facilitates Communities of Practice (CoPs) on topics such as implementation and project management, workflow redesign, vendor selection and management, Meaningful Use, privacy and security, and public health. In 2012, there were over 6,600 participants in CoPs and over 200,000 views of the CoP web pages.

- Knowledge-sharing across RECs through virtual and in-person meetings and workshops to accelerate the exchange of lessons learned and best practices from on-going implementation projects. The virtual training sessions included topics related to health information exchange as well as clinical decision support and Meaningful Use stage 2 (Table 9). In total, participation in these sessions to date exceeds over 2,700.

Table 9. Virtual trainings held for RECs in 2012 by Topic and Attendees

Date	Event Topic	Number of Attendees
April 27	Clinical Summaries Part 1: Overview	109
May 11	How to Get Burning Issues Answered	78
May 18	P&S: Recent Developments and FAQ	166
May 25	Clinical Summaries Part 2: Implementation	149
June 1	Sustainability Through Helping Specialists	167
June 8	Exchanging Key Clinical Quality Information	96
June 15	CyberSecure (Security Game Demo)	124
June 22	Health Literacy and EHR Implementation	105
July 13	Million Hearts	105
July 27	Clinical Quality Measures (Part 1)	126
August 10	Public Health Update: Immunization Reporting	105
August 24	Med Reconciliation	122
August 31	Meaningful Use Stage 2 Overview (CMS)	182
September 7	ROI Tool Demo	102
September 14	PopHealth	70
September 28	Meaningful Use Stage 2: Part 2	127
October 5	Incentive Program Tool	99
October 12	Clinical Decision Support & CQMs Part 1	105
October 19	Mobile Device Security	83
October 26	Clinical Decision Support & CQMs Part 2	80
November 2	HITRC Meaningful Use Resources	90
November 9	Stage 2 in the Workplace	87
November 16	Basics of Data Encryption	79
December 7	Broadband – Critical Access Hospitals	73
December 14	Achieving More Robust Patient & Family Engagement through Stage 2 Objectives: Using Secure Electronic Messaging Effectively	82
	Total Number of Participants	2,711

SOURCE: REC Program Data

Customer Relationship Management Tool

The REC Program uses implementation of an online Customer Relationship Management (CRM) tool to help REC and ONC monitor provider progress in EHR Incentive Programs implementation. Key accomplishments in 2012 related specifically to addressing barriers to EHR adoption include:

- Helped RECs to collect data on over 143,000 providers within the CRM to track key milestones and other information related to EHR adoption and Meaningful Use progress.

- Developed an integrated report that merges Medicare and Medicaid EHR Incentive Programs' data with the CRM data. These reports are used by RECs and other stakeholders to improve their services and monitor the success of providers as they move through the program.

- Established functionality and analytical framework to track barriers that practices are facing as they work towards achieving Meaningful Use. This has allowed ONC to take REC feedback about barriers beyond the realm of anecdotal evidence and into concrete lessons-learned from the field that can then be used to focus ONC's policy and program efforts. ONC aggregates these data nationally to identify the challenges faced by providers and guide HITRC and NLC efforts to develop solutions (Table 10).

Table 10. Top Ten Challenges Identified by Providers and Addressed by the REC Program

Type of Challenge	Overall Rank
Provider engagement	1
Meaningful Use Measures	2
Administrative practice issues (Paperwork/Planning/Merger)	3
Vendor Selection	4
Practice workflow adoption	5
Vendor delays in Implementation/Installation	6
Practice financial issues	7
Practice staff training	8
Medicaid technical issues	9
Technical vendor issues	10

SOURCE: Customer Relationship Management (CRM) Tool, maintained by the Office of Provider Adoption and Support (OPAS) at ONC, December 5, 2012.

The RECs use the CRM tool to track specific site-level challenges that practices are facing as they work towards achieving Meaningful Use. Different types of practices and providers face very different types of challenges to EHR adoption (Figure 24). For example, health centers face more difficulties with administrative issues, such as finding resources for EHR adoption among competing projects and initiatives, and workflow redesign that will allow the coordination of multiple provider types. Small private practices on the other hand, tend to have more difficulty with provider engagement and buy-in. The HITRC Communities of Practice develop mitigation strategies to address these challenges. Finally, reported challenges on specific Meaningful Use measures are used to develop strategies and educational materials.

Figure 24. Top 5 Challenges to Meaningful Use by Practice Type

Rank	CHCs	CAHs	Other Underserved Setting	Practice Consortium	Private Practice 1-10	Public Hospitals	Rural Health Clinic	Rural Hospital	Specialty Practice
1	Practice Administrative (n=329 site-level reports)	Practice Administrative (n=79)	MU Measures (n=374)	MU Measures (n=124)	Provider engagement (n=1,226)	Provider engagement (n=262)	Provider engagement (n=76)	Workflow adoption (n=123)	Practice Training (n=30)
2	MU Measures (n=294)	MU Measures (n=73)	Practice Administrative (n=121)	Practice Administrative (n=112)	MU Measures (n=964)	Practice Administrative (n=112)	Practice Administrative (n=70)	Practice Administrative (n=80)	Provider Engagement (n=16)
3	Workflow adoption (n=145)	Practice financial issues (n=69)	Provider engagement (n=109)	Workflow adoption (n=94)	Practice Administrative (n=591)	MU Measures (n=108)	Practice financial issues (n=57)	MU Measures (n=60)	MU Measures (n=14)
4	Vendor delays in Implementation/Installation (n=135)	Practice staffing (n=58)	Workflow adoption (n=105)	Vendor selection (n=80)	Vendor selection (n=587)	Vendor delays in Implementation/Installation (n=65)	MU Measures (n=50)	Provider engagement (n=14)	Vendor selection (n=12)
5	Medicaid program not set up yet (n=87)	Vendor delays in Implementation/Installation (n=45)	Vendor delays in Implementation/Installation (n=94)	Vendor upgrade (n=46)	Workflow adoption (n=449)	Vendor selection (n=58)	Vendor selection (n=43)	Vendor delays in Implementation/Installation (n=13)	Workflow adoption (n=11)

MU Measures	Attestation Process	Practice Issue	Vendor Issue

SOURCE: Customer Relationship Management (CRM) Tool, maintained by the Office of Provider Adoption and Support (OPAS) at ONC, December 5, 2012.

ADDRESSING BARRIERS TO EHR ADOPTION RELATED TO PRIVACY & SECURITY OF ELECTRONIC HEALTH INFORMATION

As noted in the section describing the efforts Office of the Chief Privacy Officer related to adoption, ONC has undertaken several key initiatives to undertake address privacy and security concerns, which may affect provider adoption and implementation of EHRs. In addition to providing education and outreach, OCPO also addresses specific potential vulnerabilities and capabilities to provide consumers greater control over their health information, as described below.

Education & Outreach regarding Best Practices regarding Privacy & Security. In response to grantee and other stakeholder concerns, and to requests for plain language materials regarding privacy and security best practices, ONC, in coordination with OCR, develops policies and toolkits that help vendors, providers, and consumers adopt and utilize health IT privacy and security.

- OCPO developed privacy and security-oriented technical assistance materials for ONC grantees and other stakeholders, including a cybersecurity video game to help providers train their employees on general security practices to safeguard ePHI, and a variety of resources addressing the security of ePHI when using mobile devices, including videos, fact sheets and other downloadable resources. Hosted on ONC's public website, www.HealthIT.gov, and linked to other stakeholders' websites, these interactive modules will depict various real-world scenarios involving potential security breaches of patient health information.

- OCPO reviewed the Health IT Policy Committee recommendations on privacy and security safeguards and health information exchange, particularly those with respect to affording individuals' the choice of whether to participate in certain types of electronic health information exchange, and furthered the adoption of these recommendations through the release of the State HIE Privacy and Security Program Instruction Notice to grantees.

- In 2013, ONC is researching innovative ways to identify barriers to consumer understanding of how providers may use and disclose protected health information about their patients as explained in a notice of privacy practices for protected health information, which is required to be distributed to patients by the HIPAA Privacy Rule. Such usability research will help to further refine and modify specific features of the wording and/or presentation formats to maximize communication effectiveness.

Health Information Breaches. In response to health care providers' increased adoption of mobile devices such as laptops, smart phones and computer tablets for delivering health care, the Office of the OCPO and the Health IT Policy Committee (HITPC) identified lost and stolen unencrypted mobile devices as a major source of health information breaches. ONC undertook several key initiatives to address this vulnerability:

- OCPO, in conjunction with the HHS Office for Civil Rights (OCR), hosted a successful (1,000+ participants) public roundtable and comment period on securing and protecting health information while using mobile devices across various health care delivery settings. The result of the roundtable and the public comment period was the development and release of an educational initiative and resource center for those in the clinical sector on how to protect and secure health information when using a mobile device.

- OCPO developed testing protocols to analyze popular mobile devices (smart phones, tablets, and laptop computers) to determine security measures needed to keep health information secured on mobile devices. This resulted in the development of:

    o An assessment of mobile devices currently on the market to determine if they have security features built in that would assist in compliance with NIST and HITECH standards that an individual could manually enable "out of the box" to protect health information accessed or stored on the device.

    o Suggested ways to configure the devices to improve "out of the box" security. These device-specific guidelines will soon be publicly available on HealthIT.gov

- In FY 2012, OCPO engaged in data gathering activities to further identify the issues surrounding mobile health by conducting a series of focus groups to identify and explore consumer attitudes, concerns and preferences on the privacy and security of health-related information communicated via mobile devices in. In FY 2013, ONC plans to release a report on this information and share results.

Greater Patient Control and Choice. Because exchanging a patient's health information electronically may increase the risk of revealing information a patient did not want to share, there is a desire for electronic systems to have the capability to capture patient choice and subsequently "segment" the information on a granular level to reflect the patient's wishes. The lack of this capability in current systems is viewed as an implementation barrier. To address this, ONC funded pilots to demonstrate the feasibility of proposed privacy and security policy solutions related to this concern.

- OCPO provided ongoing management of the Strategic Health IT Advanced Research Project for Security (SHARP-S) grant, which encompasses a series of research projects focused on the following areas: Audit Management, Integrity Management, Media Management, Access Management, and Security Program Management. The privacy and security solutions developed under the SHARP-S grant are intended to move the marketplace forward and inform policy development.

- OCPO initiated an eConsent pilot project to develop, pilot, and evaluate innovative ways to meaningfully inform individuals of their choices regarding sharing of their electronic health information and to electronically capture the individuals' choice.

- OCPO supported the Data Segmentation for Privacy Initiative (DS4P), which is working across the federal space and with industry partners to identify innovative ways of protecting the privacy of health information. Sharing a patient's health information electronically may increase the risk that information is sent that a patient did not want to share. ONC launched and completed an initiative through the S&I framework to explore the ability of EHRs to "segment" health information (*i.e.,* isolate and send only specific parts of a medical record). Through the participation of a diverse group of stakeholders (including VA and SAMSHA), the initiative identified current standards that could be used to "tag" sensitive information protected by law or patient choices, and the pilots demonstrated that these standards could be implemented in an EHR.

- OCPO is also supporting a study regarding the provenance of data in PHRs, EHRs, and health information exchange organizations' data stores, conducting a landscape assessment of how such entities currently track the provenance of clinical information within their systems, and determining whether there are gaps preventing these systems from producing and sharing that information in a clinical document.

BARRIERS TO ADOPTION AMONG PROVIDERS INELIGIBLE FOR THE EHR INCENTIVE PROGRAM

Similar to office-based physicians, behavioral health care providers' top barriers relate to costs— upfront and ongoing maintenance costs.[37] Lack of skilled staff to select, implement, and maintain systems are other key barriers, in addition to provider resistance and privacy laws. A number of challenges have been identified with regards to health IT adoption in long-term and post-acute care settings, including differences in clinical processes and information needs; lack of staff, leadership and organizational skills and capacity to acquire, implement and use technology; and lack of awareness of and need for interoperable HIE solutions.[38]

EFFORTS TO ENABLE BEHAVIORAL HEALTH IT

ONC convened a day-long Behavioral Health IT Roundtable to help develop a behavioral health IT strategy that could enable enhanced coordination and integration of primary care and behavioral health.[39] Key areas where heath IT was identified as having the potential to enhance greater integration between primary care and behavioral include: care coordination; patient engagement; medication management, adherence and abuse; and streamline and standardize reporting.

Health IT solutions are being developed to reduce prescription drug misuse and overdose by increasing access to state-run electronic databases (known as Prescription Drug Monitoring Programs (PDMPs) used to track the prescribing and dispensing of controlled prescription drugs to patients.[40,41] PDMP data is intended to enhance healthcare providers' understanding of their patients' prescription drug history and support clinical decision-making. Despite their clinical usefulness, evidence suggests that PDMPs are underutilized because they are difficult to access.

The *Enhancing Access to Prescription Drug Monitoring Programs using Health Information Technology* project, funded by the Substance Abuse and Mental Health Services Administration (SAMHSA) and managed by ONC in partnership with the SAMHSA, Centers for Disease Control and Prevention, and the Office of National Drug Control Policy, involved launching pilots to demonstrate the viability of real-time, electronic coordination among PDMPs and ambulatory care providers, emergency department providers, pharmacists, and opioid treatment program providers. The pilots demonstrated that using health IT could improve healthcare providers' ability to access important PDMP data at the point of care. To implement these pilots, ONC developed various technology solutions for exchanging PDMP data and electronically incorporating this information directly into clinical workflows.

In order to enhance coordination and integration of primary care and behavioral health, SAMHSA and ONC collaborated to jointly develop and electronically specify behavioral health clinical quality measures to be added to the current portfolio of suitable measures for Meaningful Use of EHRs. An interagency workgroup on behavioral health information technology with representatives from 18 federal agencies made consensus recommendations which were accepted by the ONC HIT Policy Committee and referred to the HITPC Quality Measures Workgroup for development. Currently, ONC is putting forth consensus recommendations for Stage 3 of Meaningful Use through the Health IT Standard Committee's Implementation workgroup.

There are several initiatives that seek to address the challenges associated with diversity of privacy regulations at the state and federal level governing behavioral health data exchange. In 2012, the SAMHSA funded a year-long pilot project with five State HIE Program grantees (KY, IL, ME, OK, RI) to work through the challenges of exchanging substance abuse and mental health treatment data and to develop infrastructure supporting the exchange of health information among behavioral health and physical health providers. The participants worked to develop local consent policies and a common consent form that is compliant with federal requirements (42 CFR Part 2). The participating HIEs are continuing to work to implement the necessary consent management processes within their current technological infrastructure.

Additionally, ONC funded the Behavioral Health Data Exchange Consortium, which was created to pilot the interstate exchange of behavioral health treatment records among treating health care providers using the Nationwide Health Information Direct protocols. This is an activity of the State Health Policy Consortium and consists of six participating State HIE Program grantees: AL, FL, KY, NM, NE, and MI. The project involves the creation of draft policies and procedures for the exchange of behavioral health treatment records that are compliant with federal (42 CFR Part 2) and participating state mental health laws and regulations.

ONC also initiated the Data Segmentation for Privacy (DSP4) Initiative, which will enable the implementation and management of more complex disclosure policies. This project develops and tests standards for managing patient consent and data segmentation (*e.g.,* enable the sharing of some but not all health information) that can specifically enable behavioral health data exchange though could be adopted across different types of providers. An implementation guide for consent management and data segmentation was released in the summer of 2012. SAMHSA and the VA are collaborating on an initial test implementation of these standards and currently there are three ongoing pilot projects.

EFFORTS TO ENABLE HEALTH IT AMONG LONG-TERM AND POST-ACUTE CARE PROVIDERS

A recent ONC report describes many of the issues related to health IT in long-term and post-acute care settings.[42] ONC has undertaken several efforts to support health IT adoption among long-term and post-acute care providers. ONC convened a day-long roundtable with stakeholders to assess the specific needs for EHR and HIE services among LTPAC providers and make LTPAC providers aware of EHR system features and functions that could help support transitions of care, care coordination, and related HIE functions.[43] ONC's State HIE Program has also provided assistance to 21 states to address exchange disparities among long-term care facilities. The State HIE program has set up a Community of Practice for LTPAC which convenes State HIE grantees and other federal grantees interested in working on LTPAC care coordination and transition in care problems that can be addressed through HIE by sharing knowledge and experience, translating learning into practice, and fostering relationships that can enable real-world implementation.

Additionally, in February 2011, ONC awarded ten Challenge Grants intended "to encourage breakthrough innovations for health information exchange and interoperability."[44] Four State HIE Program grantees (Colorado, Maryland, Massachusetts, and Oklahoma) were each awarded approximately $1.7 million to improve long-term and post acute care (LTPAC) transitions. The grantees have identified strategies and approaches that can be widely adopted by communities seeking to improve transitions of care to and from LTPAC providers, including:

- Common processes and appropriate connection points for clinical information transfer between hospitals and LTPAC providers

- Recommendations for hospital and LTPAC provider data needs

- Strategies to promote the use of standards based technology to create, transmit and view clinical documents of relevance to LTPAC

- Approaches to engage LTPAC providers where they are today across the health IT adoption spectrum (from high adoption to no adoption)

ONC has also sought to identify opportunities for long-term and post-acute care (LTPAC) providers to use health IT to enable care coordination, remote monitoring to support at home care, and tools to support care planning and managing care across the continuum of care.[45]

Additionally, ONC's S&I Framework activities extend beyond advancing HIE for only professionals eligible for financial incentive payments through the EHR Incentive Programs. One specific example includes the Longitudinal Coordination of Care Workgroup, a community-led initiative with multiple public and private sector individuals, each committed to overcoming interoperability challenges in long-term, post-acute care (LTPAC) transitions. In collaboration with support and funding by the Office of the Assistant Secretary for Planning and Evaluation (ASPE), this workgroup supports and advances interoperable HIE on behalf of LTPAC stakeholders and promotes care coordination on behalf of medically-complex and/or functionally impaired persons. Its primary goal is to identify standards that support care coordination of medically-complex and/or functionally impaired persons that are aligned with and could be included in the EHR Incentive Programs. The Workgroup consists of two active sub-workgroups:

1) Longitudinal Care Plan, focused on the identification of standards for an interoperable, longitudinal care plan, including the home health plan of care, which aligns, supports and informs patient-centric care delivery across the care continuum; and

2) LTPAC transitions, focused on the identification of data elements for LTPAC transitions of care and care plan information exchange. Stakeholders interested in participating in the workgroup, providing feedback, or piloting emerging standards are encouraged to participate.[46]

BARRIERS TO HEALTH INFORMATION EXCHANGE

Currently, there is limited sharing of health information during transitions of care among providers.[47] A 2012 Commonwealth Fund survey of U.S. primary care physicians found that less than one in four physicians is notified when their patient visits the emergency room and less than half receive information needed to help manage their patient's care within 48 hours after discharged from the hospital. Furthermore, only 16 percent receive information from specialists regarding changes made to their patient's medication or care plan.

Increasing providers' capability to electronically exchange information with other providers has the potential to help address existing gaps in health information sharing between health care providers. Providers overwhelmingly believe that electronic health information has the potential to improve the quality of patient care and coordinate care.[48] Expanding interoperability can make it easier and less costly to share health information among providers.

ONC recognizes that increasing electronic exchange of health information among providers will involve a multi-pronged approach. Some key challenges perceived by physicians relate to technical barriers, such as the ability of EHR systems to communicate with other systems, the lack of an exchange infrastructure, and the costs of exchanging health information, such as interface costs and transaction fees.[49] In addition to concerns regarding costs and interoperability of EHR systems, providers may not be aware of available mechanisms to electronically exchange health information, including state and local HIE efforts.[50] Furthermore, given that many providers do not currently share health information with other providers during transitions of care, changing providers' practice patterns or workflow is also needed to increase the electronic exchange of health information—which can be difficult. Thus, the challenge of expanding interoperable health information exchange not only lies with technology adoption and availability of needed health IT standards, but with the alignment of the service delivery and payment systems to support health information exchange.

ONC's seeks to enable exchange by:

- Providing mechanisms to exchange health information electronically;

- Expanding interoperability of systems;

- Reducing the cost and complexity of electronic health information exchange;

- Ensuring trust among the key participants of exchange; and

- Encouraging exchange of health information amongst providers, particularly during transitions of care.

ONC has been working closely with states to ensure providers have mechanisms to exchange health information electronically with other providers. As noted in the section describing the State HIE Program efforts, 39 states and territories have operational directed exchange mechanisms broadly available for providers to subscribe to statewide and 25 states have query-based exchange available statewide to providers through either a single or through multiple query services/entities.

Electronic health information exchange is a central component of the next stage of EHR Incentive Programs' Meaningful Use requirements. As part of Stage 2 of the EHR Incentive Programs, CMS introduced core requirements related to exchange that will facilitate the exchange of key clinical information during transitions of care and ensure that providers can exchange information with others, regardless of EHR vendor. These requirements should lead to advances in the technical capabilities of EHRs to exchange critical clinical information across vendor platforms, and make electronic health information exchange a priority among providers.

In addition to addressing technological barriers to exchange, CMS and ONC, working with federal partners and industry representatives, are playing a central role in trying to address a broader set of barriers relating to the "business case" of exchange. ONC, working with CMS, is trying to identify how service delivery and payment systems can encourage and support health information exchange. Specifically, ONC and CMS are pursuing another key mechanism to encourage providers to exchange information. A recent Request for Information (RFI)[xi] seeks specific suggestions from industry, health care providers, and other stakeholders on how to expand interoperability, including using a combination of incentives, payment adjustments, and requirements that will lead to a more coordinated, value-driven health care system. According to the Bipartisan Policy Center, the new Stage 2 Meaningful Use EHR Incentive Programs requirements related to health information exchange, together with new delivery system and payment models, are increasingly creating the "business case" for clinicians, hospitals, and other providers to begin sharing data electronically across organizational boundaries.[51]

State HIE Program grantees are also trying to engage health care providers and increase awareness of available options to exchange health information electronically. A case study of five states shows that states' approaches to engage providers varies as does their success in making providers more aware of their options to exchange clinical information electronically.[52] Some states plan to launch campaigns to raise awareness among small providers, while others have decided to target large health systems to increase awareness by reaching a critical mass of providers that will encourage small providers to follow suit. At a national-level, ONC developed a grantee recognition program to highlight progress to increase provider awareness. This program includes press releases templates that can help raise awareness among providers within the grantees' jurisdiction. ONC also created a variety of promotional materials, including videos and handouts that grantees can use as a communication vehicle to help demonstrate the value of HIE to providers and other stakeholders.

While larger health systems and providers may be pursuing a variety of available mechanisms to exchange health information, including private HIEs or shared technology platforms with other affiliated providers, a key role of State HIE Program grantees is to enable services to providers lacking such options. The case study of five states conducted by independent evaluators of the State HIE Program reported that each of these states has been focused on enabling services for providers that may not have other options for HIE, particularly small and rural providers. For example, Texas and Wisconsin are enabling the use of Direct Project services (which enables point-to-point exchange of health information) for small rural providers and critical access hospitals. Leadership in each of these states continues to seek ways to provide value to entities

---

[xi] https://www.federalregister.gov/articles/2013/03/07/2013-05266/advancing-interoperability-and-health-information-exchange

whose immediate exchange needs are already satisfied from non-grantee enabled services. This includes providing services, such as those that relate to public health which are not currently available. For example, some states are facilitating public health reporting for hospital systems. HIN in Maine is assisting with the electronic exchange of reportable lab results between hospitals and the public health department, while NeHII in Nebraska is also planning to offer public health reporting functionality in subsequent phases of their implementation.

ONC has also undertaken other initiatives to address some barriers related to cost and interoperability. ONC launched the Exemplar Health Information Exchange Governance Entities Program. This program will allow ONC to work with existing governance entities to further develop and adopt policies, interoperability requirements, and business practice criteria that align with national priorities. By advancing and further developing existing health information exchange governance models, this program promises to increase the level of secure electronic health information exchange in the nation, reduce the cost and complexity of implementation, and assure the privacy and security of the electronic exchange of health information.

To address the costs associated with exchanging health information electronically, State HIE Program grantees have taken a variety of responses.[53] Washington State introduced a tiered subscription model rewarding early adopters and charging subscription fees based on organization size. In addition, they attempt to maintain low operating and administrative costs to lower subscription fees. Maine has experienced high costs at the vendor level. As a result, the state has pursued relationships with multiple HIE vendors because the initial designated vendor proved to be too expensive.

ONC's continued work on developing and encouraging the adoption of standards may also help reduce the cost and complexity of exchange. The S&I Framework continues to work on various initiatives to promote standards that will increase interoperability. In 2012, a number of initiatives focused on increasing standardization, including of vocabularies used to share complex health information; the structure for sharing health information during transitions of care; the transport of health information directly from one EHR to another EHR; and the types data consumers will receive when they access their health information via Blue Button. The use of the technical standards and services comprising the Direct Project offers providers an inexpensive option to exchange health information with another provider. These and other key strategic initiatives in 2012 are described as follows:

- **Standardizing Meaning:** Federal agencies such as National Library of Medicine (NLM) at the National Institutes of Health and the National Center for Health Statistics at the Centers for Disease Control and Prevention have helped develop, support, and advance four primary vocabulary standards addressing medications (RxNorm), problem lists (SNOMED), administrative transactions (ICD-10), and laboratory test results (LOINC). The Meaningful Use requirements from the Medicare and Medicaid EHR Incentive Programs have further advanced the consistent and reproducible use of these vocabularies.

- **Standardizing Structure:** For the first time, the health IT industry has agreed upon the consolidated clinical document architecture (CCDA) as a national standard supporting transitions of care and patient care summaries. The communities that developed the consolidated CDA have taken a remarkable step to advance interoperability by creating re-usable templates and building blocks that should accelerate the use of standardized structure. As ONC continues to push for simplicity, modularity, usability, applicability, and parsimony in our health IT standards, the CCDA is a remarkable step along that path.

- **Standardizing Reporting:** A consistent national standard for public health reporting of laboratory tests, based on voluntary consensus standards – specifically, Health Level 7 (HL7) 2.5.1 standards – was adopted. While many other public health reporting standards are still used, laboratories, state and local public health agencies throughout the nation, and every certified EHR product will be able to use a clear and consistent target.

- **Standardizing Transport:** There is now a universal way to consistently and securely send information from one EHR system to another using the Direct protocol. ONC's Direct Project develops specifications for a secure, scalable, standards-based way for providers, laboratories, hospitals, pharmacies, and patients to send encrypted health information directly to known, trusted recipients over the Internet (Direct addresses are analogous to e-mail). This "open government" initiative brought together over 200 participants from more than 60 companies and organizations to assemble consensus standards that support secure exchange of basic clinical information and public health data between known and trusted providers.

- **Standardizing Access:** The Blue Button initiatives have made it possible for millions of veterans and people with Medicare to gain access to their health information. Now the community is working on standardizing the health care information that the Blue Button provides (based on the CCDA) and expanding Blue Button to include other kinds of data like financial and billing data from CMS.

- **Framework Supports Standardization Initiatives:** The S&I Framework has supported the community in initiatives that have worked on digital signatures (esMD), piloted ways to ask questions to EHRs and get consistent answers back (Query Health), created standards that can be used to share important information from hospitals and doctors' offices with long term and post-acute care providers, and explored ways of protecting parts of an electronic health record that require extra caution to assure they are not inappropriately shared (DS4P).

- **Platform to support implementation and testing:** As an extension to the S&I Framework, the Implementation and Testing (I&T) Platform launched to support the implementation and development testing of Medicare and Medicaid EHR Incentive Programs' Meaningful Use standards, and tools, examples, testing tools, and other resources needed to support achievement of interoperability and other EHR Incentive Programs' goals.

- **Supporting dissemination of CDS to enable quality improvement**: The Health eDecisions project is working to enable the broad adoption and sharable, scalable clinical decision support interventions and modules in EHRs, and completed work on its Use Case 1 – Development of Standards to structure medical knowledge in a shareable and executable format for use in CDS – in January, 2013.

- **Universal standard for transport:** In addition, in collaboration with CMS, ONC convened a multi-agency collaborative that reviewed every value set, every code and every line of logic in every EHR Incentive Programs' electronic clinical quality measure (eCQM). The partnership validated codes (SNOMED CT, Rx Norm, LOINC, etc) to ensure that every quality measure used codes that were accurate and current and logic that was consistent and unambiguous. Furthermore, all certified EHRs will report clinical quality data to fit a single standard. This standard is the Quality Reporting Document Architecture Release 2.0. The certification to this standard will enable clinical quality data to be reported to States, registries, and payers in a single consistent format.

With regards to increasing the privacy and security of electronic health information exchange, ONC's Office of the Chief Privacy Officer has also made significant efforts to help develop and encourage the adoption of policies and other key mechanisms to help ensure trusted exchange. An example of such efforts includes outlining a common set of privacy and security 'rules of the road' or guidance for State HIE Program grantees to ensure patients have the opportunity for 'meaningful choice' (either directly, or by ensuring that the providers they serve offer such choice) as to whether to participate in certain types of electronic health information exchange.

CONCLUSION

Under the HITECH Act, the CMS Medicare and Medicaid EHR Incentive Programs are designed to accelerate the adoption of health IT (specifically certified EHR technology) and its role in delivering high quality and affordable care. This report serves as an update for policy makers on the status of adoption and the progress of CMS and ONC programs in helping to establish a nationwide system for electronic use and exchange of health information.

Since the passage of the HITECH Act, there had been substantial growth in adoption of EHRs and other EHR technology related to Meaningful Use requirements from the EHR Incentive Programs, which has the potential to improve our nation's health. Eligible professionals and hospitals are making incredible progress towards attaining Meaningful Use. Specifically:

★ In 2012, nearly three-quarters of office-based physicians (72 percent) had adopted any EHR system. Forty percent of physicians have adopted a "basic" EHR with certain advanced capabilities, more than double the adoption rate in 2009. Physician adoption rates for 12 of the fifteen Meaningful Use requirements for the Medicare and Medicaid EHR Incentive Programs' Stage 1 core objectives were at least fifty percent.

★ As of 2012, 44 percent of non-federal acute care hospitals had adopted a "basic" EHR, more than triple the adoption rate of 2009. The percent of hospitals possessing certified EHR technology increased by 18 percent between 2011 and 2012, rising from 72 percent to 85 percent. Hospital adoption rates for Meaningful Use Stage 1 requirements for the EHR Incentive Programs' ranged from 72 percent to 94 percent.

★ The percent of physicians e-prescribing using an EHR on one of the nation's largest e-prescribing network (Surescripts) increased almost eight-fold from 7 percent in December 2008 to over half of physicians (54 percent) in December 2012. In the same period, the percent of community pharmacies active on the Surescripts network grew from 69 percent to 95 percent. The percent of new and renewal prescriptions sent electronically between 2008 and 2012 has increased ten-fold to approximately 47 percent.

• As of April 2013, more than 291,000 professionals, representing more than half of the nation's eligible professionals, have received incentive payments through the EHR Incentive Programs. Over 3,800 hospitals, including CAHs, representing about 80 percent of eligible hospitals, which include CAHs, have received incentive payments through this program as well.

• As of January 1, 2013, the 62 RECs are actively working with close to 132,000 primary care providers and more than 11,000 specialists to achieve Meaningful Use by 2014, surpassing the 2012 HHS High Priority Goal of providing assistance to 100,000 primary care providers.

• A GAO report found that Medicare providers working with a REC were over 2.3 times more likely to receive a Medicare EHR Incentive Payment then those who weren't working with an REC. The RECs are also working with over 1,164 critical access and other small hospitals that have 50 beds or less, which is approximately 67 percent of the practices of this size in the Country. Of the CAH/RH working with RECs, 19 percent achieved Meaningful Use by the end of 2013.

CMS' and ONC's programs and offices have played a central role in supporting the widespread adoption of health IT, including identifying and addressing barriers to the adoption and Meaningful Use of EHRs. CMS and ONC will continue to address challenges related to HIE and build on the efforts of the State HIE Program to offer mechanisms by which providers can exchange key clinical information.

As both public and private payers take concrete steps to change the incentives for paying providers, health IT can provide the infrastructure and the data analytics necessary to improved care coordination, better quality, and lower costs. Continued adoption of EHRs and health IT can enable the transformation of health care delivery in order to reduce health care costs and improve the well-being of Americans.

Notes

[1] Medicare and Medicaid Programs; Electronic Health Record Incentive Program; Final Rule, 75 Fed. Reg. 44,314 (July 28, 2010).

[2] Blumenthal D. Launching HITECH. N Engl J Med. 2010 Feb 4;362(5):382-5. Epub 2009 Dec 30.

[3] Blumenthal D. Launching HITECH. N Engl J Med. 2010 Feb 4;362(5):382-5. Epub 2009 Dec 30.

[4] Buntin MB, Jain SH, Blumenthal D. Health information technology: laying the infrastructure for national health reform. Health Aff (Millwood). 2010 Jun;29(6):1214-9.

[5] Adoption of "Basic" electronic health records as defined in: Hsiao CJ, et al. Electronic Medical Record/Electronic Health Record Systems of Non-hospital-based physicians: United States, 2009 and Preliminary 2010 State Estimates Health E Stats. National Center for Health Statistics, Centers for Disease Control. Source: National Center for Health Statistics, Centers for Disease Control, NAMC (National Ambulatory Medical Care) Survey (mail-only respondents), 2008-2010

[6] King J, Patel V, Furukawa MF. Physician Adoption of Electronic Health Record Technology to Meet Meaningful Use Objectives: 2009-2012. ONC Data Brief, no. 7. Washington, DC: Office of the National Coordinator for Health Information Technology. December 2012.

[7] Basic EHR adoption requires the EHR system to have at least a basic set of EHR functions, including clinician notes, as defined Jha et al. Jha AK, DesRoches CM, Campbell EG, Donelan K, Rao SR, Ferris TG, et al. Use of electronic health records in U.S. hospitals. N Engl J Med. 2009; 360(16):1628-38.

[8] A certified EHR is EHR technology that has been certified as meeting federal requirements for some or all of the hospital objectives of Meaningful Use. Possession means that the hospital has a legal agreement with the EHR vendor, but is not equivalent to adoption.

[9] Charles D, King J, Patel V, Furukawa MF. "Adoption of Electronic Health Record Systems among U.S. Non-federal Acute Care Hospitals: 2008-2012," ONC Data Brief, no 9. Washington, DC: Office of the National Coordinator for Health Information Technology. March 2013.

[10] Updated ONC analysis of Surescripts data. Hufstader M, Swain M, Furukawa MF. State Variation in E-Prescribing Trends in the United States. ONC Data Brief, no. 4. Washington, DC: Office of the National Coordinator for Health Information Technology, November 2012.

[11] Medicare and Medicaid Programs; Electronic Health Record Incentive Program; Final Rule, 75 Fed. Reg. 44,314 (July 28, 2010). http://www.cms.gov/Regulations-and-Guidance/Legislation/EHRIncentivePrograms/Meaningful_Use.html

[12] National Center for Health Statistics. National Ambulatory Medical Care Survey: Physician Workflow Supplement, 2011.

[13] Hsiao CJ, Hing E. Use and characteristics of electronic health record systems among office-based physician practices: United States, 2001–2012. NCHS data brief, no 111. Hyattsville, MD: National Center for Health Statistics. 2012.

[14] Charles D, King J, Patel V, Furukawa MF. "Adoption of Electronic Health Record Systems among U.S. Non-federal Acute Care Hospitals: 2008-2012," ONC Data Brief, no 9. Washington, DC: Office of the National Coordinator for Health Information Technology. March 2013.

[15] Health information technology in the United States: Where we stand, 2008. Robert Wood Johnson Foundation. 2008

[16] King J, Patel V, Furukawa MF. Physician Adoption of Electronic Health Record Technology to Meet Meaningful Use Objectives: 2009-2012. ONC Data Brief, no. 7. Washington, DC: Office of the National Coordinator for Health Information Technology. December 2012.

[17] Charles D, King J, Furukawa MF, Patel V. "Hospital Adoption of Electronic Health Record Technology to Meet Meaningful Use Objectives: 2008-2012," ONC Data Brief, no. 10. Washington, DC: Office of the National Coordinator for Health Information Technology. March 2013

[18] National Council for Community Behavioral Healthcare. HIT Adoption and Readiness for Meaninful Use in Community Behavioral Health: Report on the 2012 National Council Survey. 2012. Accessed May 13, 2013 from: http://www.thenationalcouncil.org/galleries/business-practice%20files/HIT%20Survey%20Full%20Report.pdf

[19] National Center for Health Statistics. National Study for Long-Term Care Providers. 2011. Accessed May 13, 2013 from: http://www.cdc.gov/nchs/data/nsltcp/NSLTCP_FS.pdf

[20] Holup AA, Dobbs D, Meng H, Hyer K. Facility characteristics associated with the use of electronic health records in residential care facilities. J Am Med Inform Assoc. 2013 May 3. [Epub ahead of print]

[21] Centers for Disease Control and Prevention. Adoption of Health Information Technology among U.S. Ambulatory and Long-term Care Providers. Accessed May 15, 2013. http://www.cdc.gov/nchs/ppt/nchs2012/SS-03_HSIAO.pdf

[22] Wolf L, Harvell J, Jha AK. Hospitals ineligible for federal meaningful-use incentives have dismally low rates of adoption of electronic health records, Health Affairs. 2012 Mar;31(3):505-13

[23] Hufstader M, Swain M, Furukawa MF. State Variation in E-Prescribing Trends in the United States. ONC Data Brief, no. 4. Washington, DC: Office of the National Coordinator for Health Information Technology, November 2012.

[24] Friedman MA, Schueth A, Bell DS. Interoperable Electronic Prescribing In The United States: A Progress Report. Health Aff (Millwood). 2009;28(2):393-403.

[25] Surescripts. National Progress Report on e-Prescribing and Safe-Rx Rankings. 2012. Accessed May 8, 2013 from: http://www.surescripts.com/downloads/npr/National%20Progress%20Report%20on%20E%20Prescribing%20Year%202012.pdf

[26] Medicare and Medicaid Programs; Electronic Health Record Incentive Program; Final Rule, 75 Fed. Reg. 44,314 (July 28, 2010). http://www.cms.gov/Regulations-and-Guidance/Legislation/EHRIncentivePrograms/Meaningful_Use.html

[27] GAO, *Electronic Health Records: Number and Characteristics of Providers Awarded Medicare Incentive Payments for 2011*, GAO-12-778R (Washington, D.C.: July 26, 2012).

[28] Samuel CA, King J, Adetosoye F, Samy L, Furukawa MF. Engaging providers in underserved areas to adopt electronic health records. *American Journal of Managed Care*. 2013;19(3):229-34.

[29] Heisey-Grove D, Hawkins K, Jones E, Shanks K, Lynch K. Supporting Health Information Technology Adoption in Federally Qualified Health Centers. ONC Data Brief, no. 8. Washington, DC: Office of the National Coordinator for Health Information Technology, February, 2013.

[30] Heisey-Grove D, Hufstader M, Hollin I, Samy L, Shanks, K. Progress towards the meaningful use of electronic health records among critical access and small rural hospitals working with Regional Extension Centers. ONC Data Brief, no. 5. Washington, DC: Office of the National Coordinator for Health Information Technology, November 2012.

[31] Heisey-Grove D, Hawkins K, Jones E, Shanks K, Lynch K. Supporting Health Information Technology Adoption in Federally Qualified Health Centers. ONC Data Brief, no. 8. Washington, DC: Office of the National Coordinator for Health Information Technology, February, 2013..

[32] http://www.informationweek.com/healthcare/leadership/blumenthal-tear-down-e-health-barriers/229204227

[33] Swain M, Vibbert D, Furukawa MF. ONC's Community College Program Trains Over 12,000 Health IT Professionals. ONC Data Brief, no. 3. Washington, DC: Office of the National Coordinator for Health Information Technology, May 2012.

[34] United States Department of Labor. Accessed May 2, 2013 from: http://www.dol.gov/opa/media/press/eta/eta20111453.htm

[35] Charles D, Bean C, Purnell-Saunders S, Furukawa MF. "Vendors of Certified Electronic Health Record Technology: Trends and Distributions from Meaningful Use Attestations as of October 31, 2012" ONC Data Brief, no 6. Washington, DC: Office of the National Coordinator for Health Information Technology. October 2012

[36] The Office of the National Coordinator for Health Information Technology (ONC). Federal Health Information Technology Strategic Plan 2011-2015. Retrieved May 9, 2013: From: http://www.healthit.gov/sites/default/files/utility/final-federal-health-it-strategic-plan-0911.pdf

[37] National Council for Community Behavioral Healthcare. HIT Adoption and Readiness for Meaninful Use in Community Behavioral Health: Report on the 2012 National Council Survey. 2012. Accessed May 13, 2013 from: http://www.thenationalcouncil.org/galleries/business-practice%20files/HIT%20Survey%20Full%20Report.pdf

[37] The Office of the National Coordinator for Health IT. Issue Brief: Health IT in Long-term and Post Acute Care. 2013. Accessed May 13, 2013 from: http://www.healthit.gov/sites/default/files/pdf/HIT_LTPAC_IssueBrief031513.pdf

[38] Ibid.

[39] The Office of the National Coordinator for Health IT. Summary Report of Findings: Behavioral Health Roundtable. 2012. Accessed May 13, 2013 from: http://www.healthit.gov/sites/default/files/bh-roundtable-findings-report_0.pdf

[40] The Office of the National Coordinator for Health IT. Linking PDMPs to Health IT. Accessed May 15, 2013 from: http://www.healthit.gov/PDMP

[41] The Office of the National Coordinator for Health IT. Use of Health Information Technology to Optimize Provider Access and Use of Prescription Drug Monitoring Information. Accessed May 15, 2013 from: http://www.healthit.gov/sites/default/files/aspa_0126_onc_fs_pdmp_rx_misuse_project.pdf

[42] The Office of the National Coordinator for Health IT. Issue Brief: Health IT in Long-term and Post Acute Care. 2013. Accessed May 13, 2013 from: http://www.healthit.gov/sites/default/files/pdf/HIT_LTPAC_IssueBrief031513.pdf

[43] The Office of the National Coordinator for Health IT. Summary Report: Long-Term and Post-Acute Care (LTPAC) Roundtable: http://www.healthit.gov/sites/default/files/pdf/LTPACroundtablesummary.pdf

[44] The Office of the National Coordinator for Health IT. Health Information Exchange Challenge Grant Program. Accessed May 13, 2013 from: http://www.healthit.gov/providers-professionals/health-information-exchange-challenge-grant-program

[45] The Office of the National Coordinator for Health IT. Issue Brief: Health IT in Long-term and Post Acute Care. 2013. Accessed May 13, 2013 from: http://www.healthit.gov/sites/default/files/pdf/HIT_LTPAC_IssueBrief031513.pdf

[46] Ibid.

[47] Commonwealth Fund. Article Chartpack. Schoen C & Osborn R. The Commonwealth Fund 2012 International Health Policy Survey of Primary Care Physicians. International Symposium on Health Care Policy. November 2012. http://www.commonwealthfund.org/Publications/In-the-Literature/2012/Nov/Survey-of-Primary-Care-Doctors.aspx.

[48] Clinician Perspectives on Electronic Health Information Sharing for Transitions of Care Bipartisan Policy Center Health Information Technology Initiative. October, 2012

[49] Clinician Perspectives on Electronic Health Information Sharing for Transitions of Care Bipartisan Policy Center Health Information Technology Initiative. October, 2012

[50] Dullabh P, Hovey L, Ubri P. Case Study Synthesis: Experiences from Five States in Enabling HIE. NORC at the University of Chicago. February 2013. http://www.healthit.gov/sites/default/files/casestudysynthesisdocument_2-8-13.pdf

[51] Accelerating Electronic Information Sharing to Improve Quality and Reduce Costs in Health Care. Bipartisan Policy Center Health Information Technology Initiative. October, 2012.

[52] Dullabh P, Hovey L, Ubri P. Case Study Synthesis: Experiences from Five States in Enabling HIE. NORC at the University of Chicago. February 2013. http://www.healthit.gov/sites/default/files/casestudysynthesisdocument_2-8-13.pdf

[53] Dullabh P, Hovey L, Ubri P. Case Study Synthesis: Experiences from Five States in Enabling HIE. NORC at the University of Chicago. February 2013. http://www.healthit.gov/sites/default/files/casestudysynthesisdocument_2-8-13.pdf